CONTENTS

CONTENTS

Book Owes Its Gratitude To

Almighty, whose blessings have always been with me inspiring me to learn, grasp, cultivate and express through creative writing including fictions and poetry. He has been kind and gracious enough to make me understand Homeopathy according to my little caliber. Human being is a tiny creature with negligible existence. No birth or death can take place without God's will. This means that our knowledge about health is through His gift of natural food and natural environment. Homeopathy is a therapy that has natural powers due to their 'atom-like' contents of drugs. Homeopathy heals spiritually first and hence very near to God. Homeopathy and its amazing cures are due to His grace.

Dedication

I express my rspects to late Shri Moti Lal Ailwadi who had ample of forbearance and expertise of rise from a petty bookseller and guide his sons in the right direction. A qualified engineer by profession, he was compelled to sell books after he lost everything during partition of India. His tireless hard work and knowledge about worldly affairs remain an example as to how a man can feel elevated without riches.

I also remember his son late Shri Narinder Kumar Ailawadi who dedicated his life to the service of 'Sai Baba, Shirdi Wale' and always helped the poor in need.

Important Note

Information and advice on general medicines and prescriptions on homebased methods (desi) are not intended as replacement of medical advice. The book is not a medical manual but a general reference manual. It is not a substitute for any teatment that may have been suggested by your doctor.

If any reader has a suspicion that he or she has some medical problem, it is suggested that a competent medical help should be sought.

Thanks

To my daughter, Nilima Rawal and daughter-in-law Anuradha
Dua for their efforts to find out material for this book. I also
thank my wife Uma Dua who gave me many hints about home
made remedies on care of hair and nails. The subject is nearer
to women and many of my patients in Arya Samaj Dharmarth
Hospital, Sector 19, Faridabad and Swami Sarvdanand
Dharmarth Hospital, Gopi Colony, Faridabad made me rich in
my experiments to arrive at certain tested formulas to avoid
hair loss. I thank all them.

To Shri Tara Chand Sachdeva, Rajhans Refractories,
Dhanbad for his support to me and my wife Uma during the
times when I was posted in GSI camp Isri Bazar and Girdih of
Bihar and lived in jungle/tents (during 1966-68) where no
amenities like telephones, electricity, etc. existed. He used to
send message of my family at Delhi to me through his car
driver and take me to Dhanbad for telephone talks.

To Mrs. Leela Ailawadi, Shri Surinder Ailawadi and Shri
Ravinder Ailawadi for their co-operation in all respects to write
this book.

To Shri Lakshmi Chand, Pardhan and Shri Ashok Arya,
Mantri, of Arya Samaj, Sector -19, Faridabad for showing their
confidence in me to give my independent charge of charitable
homeopathic dispensary and support my experiments for better
healing of the poor. It is this dispensary and its six to seven
hundred patients a month that enabled me write and publish
tens of articles and four books on homeopathy.

To Dr. Bhim Sen Chowdhry and Shri Om Prakash Wadhwa
for continuous encouragement to me to write this book.

To all my colleagues who devote their services to Mahrishi
Dayanand Dharmarth Aushdhalya, Sector-19, Faridabad. In
their own modernst way, they help the poor: Dr. R.C. Aggrawal,
Dr. Protima Arora, Dr. Narender Kumar Vivek, Dr. Mukesh
Goswami, Vaid Sant Ram Goyal, Dr. Sanjeev Kumar, Shri
Krishan Kumar Bhatia, Shri Ram Ji Dubey, Shri Uma Shankar,

Shri Pawan Kumar, Shri Gopi Chand, Pandit Suresh Shastri, Shri Ram Chand Arora, Mrs. Parbha, Mrs. Santosh, Mrs. Suman, Shri Om Parkash, Shri Bihari Lal, Shri Gaya Baksh, Shri Dhani Ram, Mrs. Kamla and Mrs. Sudha.

To respected Sai Ji (Sant Kishore Ji), the great saint and head of Prem Parkash Ashram, Gopi Colony, Faridabad for his kind blessings to write this book.

Dr. Shiv Dua
M. A., D. I. Hom., HMD (London)

OTHER BOOKS BY THE AUTHOR

1. Practioner's Guide to Gall Bladder and Kidney Stones.

2. Oral Diseases.

3. Neck pain—Cervical Spondylosis.

4. Know and Solve your Thyroid Problems.

5. Nail care—A Complete Solution to your Nail Problems.

Do You . . . ?

Ever think as to why should you dye your gray hair?

Want to turn premature gray hair black, the natural way?

Want to know reasons and treatment of gray hair in children?

Want to colour hair with henna in suitable method?

Want to apply henna on the hair even when the hairs are not gray?

Want to know correct method of treatment of dandruff?

Want to remove dandruff quickly?

Want to kill head-lice without use of branded chemicals?

Want to know how women can eliminate unwanted hair on chin, face, above lips?

Want to know about falling of hair, bald spots and treatment?

Test whether you are having disease of falling of hair (alopecia)?

Want to know correct method of combing, brushing and select hair oils and shampoos?

Have no time to wash your hair today still want to have looks of hair as if washed?

Want to know that after effects of haircuts can be cured by homeopathy?

Want to know what is barber's itch?

Want to prevent allergy of hair dye or hair color?

Read on . . .

Some Facts

- The best care of hair is done with the help of home remedies.

- Rinsing hair with sour curd brings shine to hair and avoids hair falling.

- Eat those food which are rich in protein, carotenes, have essential iron, silica, zinc, vitamin B, C, E and fatty acids.

- Do not take excessive cold drinks (carbonated). These acidify the blood and starve hair of minerals.

- A cold bath stimulates the circulation of blood and aids in the in the head strengthens the hair. Water is a valuable health promoter.

- Do not tie hair-bunches too tight as done in making ponytails. Extreme tightening of hair may result in hair loss.

- Good sleep, gentle brushing and gentle combing make the hair live longer.

- Keep the hair brush and combs clean. Wash them with warm water and clean them with small steel brushes available in the market.

- Do not use combs and brushes of others and do not allow others to use your combs and brushes.

- Massaging of hairs with oil should be done regularly after or before washing the hair. It should not be with full palm-pressure but by tips of the fingers, separating the hairs at places turn-by-turn and applying oil.

- Tension makes the scalp muscles tense and prevents sufficient nutrient-blood to reach hair follicles. Starved hair roots shrink and fall out.

- Oils, shampoos, hair colors/dyes and conditioners should be selected after verifying their results from colleagues.

- Select matching products for your hair type: dry or oily.

- After washing the hair, allow them dry up naturally. Too long use of hair dryer and blowing hot air near your hair is harmful for health of hair.

- Better not to try bleaching, perm, curling, waving, use of heated rollers and winding etc. at home. Help of expert professionals should be taken for these jobs.

- In case of hair-coloring at home, follow the instructions given by manufactures. In case of dying/coloring of hairs at parlors, choose herbal products with contents like henna and other vegetable dyes.

- Dandruff or hair loss may be due to body illness, harsh cosmetics, stress, incorrect nutrition and effects of some medicines.

- Temporary hair thinning may be due to stress, shocks, childbirth, illness and ill effects of medicines.

- Hair loss at patches may be due to fungal infection like ringworm etc.

- Excessive greasyness of hair can be removed easily by rinsing hair with distilled water and lemon juice.

- Head lice can be easily removed by using wet 'nit-comb' (lice comb).

- A long with hair problems, if you have symptoms like weight loss or weariness or fatigue, better consult the doctor.

Read much more in the book . . .

Preface

Hair . . .

Since times immemorial, the care of hair, loss of hair and diseases of hair has been under strict surveillance of people of all countries and races. The concern for hair-care is much revealed in old religious books. In 'Mahabharata', when 'Dropadi's' 'sari' was unwrapped in the presence of courtesans, she vowed to rinse her hair with blood of 'Duryodhana', 'Bhim' implemented it later. In Bible, it is written, 'When a man has lost his hair and he is bald, he is clean.' There are proverbs also showing concern of hair. "Yeh Baal dhoop mien safed nahin kiye" (These hairs have not turned gray in the sun) explains experience aspect that gray hair depict. "Glory of young men is their strength, gray hair the splendor of the old." Importance of hair cannot be ignored.

Hair is most wonderful and distinctive feature of one's pesonality. If you had a hair-cut or coloured your hair, your friends would immediately notice and enquire you. You are noticed because of this crowning glory.

Hair and nails are specialized forms of keratin. Keratin is a protein found in all horny tissues. Skin, hair and nail and made of keratin. Hair has more than ninety percent of protein of a different kind that has chief content of sulphur. Chemically, keratin is not active and this is the reason, why it is capable of tolerating harsh winds, seasons and rough handling. Genetic factor and the cells, called melanocytes, decide the color of the hair. The product of melanocytes is a pigment called melanin that is found throghout the hair and skin. In judging personality of a young lad or lass, hair account for seventy percent of the total personality-count and this is the reason why people are much conscious about health of hair. Hair falling, dandruff or premature gray hair is a matter of concern for people and they start consulting elders in the home, their friends and doctors. Caring for hair is not a bad trend but the worst is to get lured to advertisements in magazines and televisions that dictate use of various brands of soaps, shampoos, oils, hair dyes and creams to erase problems of hairs. This sort of ad-invasion does more of harm than benefit. *This book guides the reader for selection of right hair-products to save your hair.*

In USA, Europe and rest of world, hair beauty is of great concern and people spend lot of money in maintaining health of hair. The emotional upset of losing hair is so much that people have organized 'Bald men' associations in order to be jovial amidst the company of fellow bald men. Use of wig is quite common in the West. If you see a lady of seventy years with shapely figure, sparkling teeth, long shining and strong hair, least wrinkled face and no spectacles, please see her in her home-privacy. Everything artificial is available, right from wigs to teeth, facial treatments to abdomen depressing gadgets and other cosmetics to suit your personality. City dwellers are much conversant with terms like threading, bleaching, facial cleaning, manicure, pedicure, head massage, leg or arm waxing and even permanent excess body hair removel by light sheer diode laser method. *Hair implantation and weaving are also common non-surgical methods for planting artificial hair on the scalp.* This book has information about these aspect as well.

In India, everyone cannot afford the cost of such beauty-luxuries but there is no dearth of money for preparing the hair on special functions like marriages and parties.

Generally, people avoid consulting a doctor in disorders like cold, cough or fever. They purchase patent medicines or cough syrups from the chemist. In the case of falling of hair or dandruff, people purchase anything on verbal advice of the chemist like cough pills, etc. In doing so, inadvertently they play havoc with the hair-health. Hair disorders are not like cold, cough or fever. *Hair relates more to diseases than disorders.* Let us understand that in some conditions, general falling of hair and dandruff can be graded as disorder due to after-effect of allergies, allopathic medicines, prolonged illness, self abuse of body (faulty diet), use of cheap cosmetics, oils and faulty care of hair. Care of hair is one aspect, which people are not fully aware of. For example, people apply oil on hair when the hair are still wet after washing or apply oil by rubbing them vigorously. Hair have to be dried properly in natural way and application of hair is gentle tapping and massaging at their roots with oiled finger-tips. Similarly frequent coloring, curling, styling and dyeing make an adverse impact on the hair. *This book has all the details about care of hair in simple language to benefit the readers.*

In some families, there is a healthy trend of well-groomed hair in all the members of family. I have enquired about this from such families and found that it is not only the hereditary blessing but the tradition of good upkeep of hair also. They thrive on habits of proper washing, drying and oiling with home made medicines. Right from the grand mothers, the proper care of hair has been given a priority. It is just like adhering to tradition of taking of 'Idli-Dosa' by South Indians, 'fish' by Bengalis and 'Rajma' by North Indians. Such life styles and food habits get developed in different regions by the climatic compulsions, local environments and agricultural produces. This also includes care of hair, diet and oil-applications. Treatment of minor diseases can be done at home without medicines. *The book has information about kitchen foods that help to restore the health of hair.*

Permanent baldness is another aspect that is dealt with in this book. *Use of wigs, hair implantation (non-surgical), hair weaving and microwefting* are detailed in the book for the general knowledge of the readers.

Premature gray hair and falling of hair are most wanting subjects of the era and it has been given adequate place in this book.

Excessive hair on the chin, cheeks and upper lips is a matter of concern for women. Treatment and method of hair removal of such hair has been adequately explained in this book.

So far as homeopathic treatment is concerned, not much of it has been mentioned except main remedies for diseases of hair. It is because the problems of hair cannot be treated at home and consultation of a doctor is required. It has been seen that homeopathic medicines show more of efficacy in treatment of both hair and nails.

Dr. Shiv Dua,
2617, Sector-16,
Faridabad 121 002
Phone: 2281764

Chapter 1

All About Hairs

All About Hair

WHAT IS HAIR?

Hair grow on the skin. They guard our skin as the skin guards our body. Hair is a bad conductor of both cold and heat. On the chest of men, hair act as a woolen garment that promotes warmth in cold weather and protects from heat in summer. During puberty when the semen starts forming in the body, it excites heat. The hair in the pubic region and under the armpits work as heat absorber. Some doctors are of the view that hair from this region should not be clean shaved and cut lengthwise.

Skin is multi-layered outer covering of our body. The uppermost layer of skin is called epidermis. Beneath this epidermis is the dermis. Epidermis is continuously shedding. Dermis is a thicker layer containing nerves, blood vessels, glands and hair follicles. Hair follicle is sebaceous gland that supplies sebum (oily substance) lubricating the skin and hair. Sebum is anti-bacterial and anti-fungal. Follicle is where the hair is born, where it lives and where it dies. It also supplies nourishment to the cells of the growing hair. The shape and size of follicle decides the life of a hair. Beneath the dermis is a layer of fatty tissue. All this is described in length in following paragraphs.

Hair are of cylindrical shape, elongated, horny formations originated from the epidermis and are planted in oblique fashion in depressions in corium known as hair follicles or hair sacs. Generally, one hair occupy only one hair sac but in some rare cases, two or even three hair come up from one sac. The ducts of the sebaceous glands open into the hair sac. Hair is composed of altered keratinized cells of cutaneous (belonging to the skin) epithelium (the cells covering all cutaneous and mucous surfaces together with the secreting cells of glands developed from ectoderm). Only the cells of the hair bulb contain no keratin (keratin—a protein found in all horny tissues). These cells continuously multiply. The hair grows from the hair bulb.

The hair that we see or the visible part of a hair is called the *shaft* and the invisible part is called *root*. The shaft is, therefore, above the skin and the root is beneath the skin. Shaft of hair is made up of keratin and is composed of dead tissues. It is because of these dead tissues that we do not feel any pain while cutting them from the stem.

The thickened part of the root is called *hair bulb.* In other words, the shaft of the hair has a root, which has a tube-like depression in the skin and it is called *follicle.* A hair sac surrounds the hair root, which contain cutaneous epithelium and connective tissue. Actually growth or development of hair is from the bottom of the follicle, called *dermal papilla.* In other words, hair bulb has a recess, which contains the papilla. Papilla (a minute nipple shaped eminence) is composed of connective tissue and contains blood capillaries that nourish the hair bulb. In case the root gets damaged, the growth of hair stops and on extreme damage, the hair may never grow.

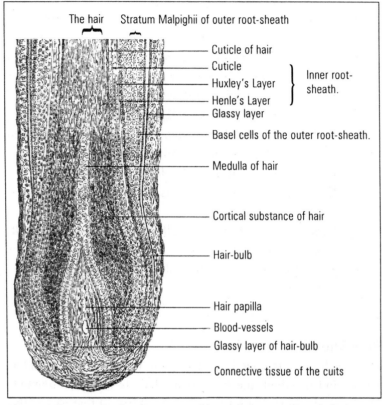

The hair   Stratum Malpighii of outer root-sheath

———— Cuticle of hair
———— Cuticle
———— Huxley's Layer   } Inner root-
———— Henle's Layer   } sheath.
———— Glassy layer
———— Basel cells of the outer root-sheath.

———— Medulla of hair

———— Cortical substance of hair

———— Hair-bulb

———— Hair papilla
———— Blood-vessels
———— Glassy layer of hair-bulb
———— Connective tissue of the cuits

Figure 1.1—Longitudinal section of human hair and its follicle.
(diagrammatic after Böhm and Davidoff; X about 300).

Anatomy of hair *(Longitudinal section wise)*

- Hair is a cylindrical shaft.
- Hair is not hollow. It is harder on the outside than in the center of the hair shaft.
- The middle part is hair.
- The middle is divided into two, like a fork at the lower end. The junction, as well as the forked ends, of the hair is called *Medulla of the hair*.
- The first layer of hair (outer) is *cuticle of hair*.

- In-between cuticle and medulla, is cortical substance of hair.
- Over cuticle is *Huxley's Layer.*
- Over Huxley's layer is *Henley's Layer.*
- Over Henley's layer is *Glassy Layer.*
- In-between the Henley's Layer and Glassy Layer, is *Stratum Malpighii* of outer root-sheath. This root sheath is wider on the stem of hair but at the forked point of·the hair root, it is thinned and runs along the fork from both sides.
- Over the root-sheath are *basal cells* of the outer root-sheath.
- Formation over basal cells all around is called *hair bulb* (lower bowl type).
- The base over which the bulb lies is *connective tissues* of the cutis.

Hair Sheaths

The hair follicle is a sac like depression in the corium as stated earlier and in which the bulb of the hair is firmly implanted. The hair follicle includes the lower two thirds of that part of the hair, which is found in the skin and the coverings of the hair is known as *hair-sheaths.* This external root sheath consists of a turning inward of the rete (net) and lines the whole follicle. It is thinnest at the base and the neck of the hair-papilla, consisting in these locations of one or two rows of cells. It is several times thicker than the root-sheath proper and is thicker at the middle of follicle. The sheath practically forms a hollow cylinder that has the hair and its envelopes.

The inner or internal root-sheath of the hair was formerly considered as divided in two layers called *Henley's and Huxley's.* Henley's layer is one cell thick and lies to the outer root sheath. Huxley's layer is two or three cells thick and lies in the middle of the sheath (See figure 1.1).

"These are not distinct layers. They are only parts of a single layer, so modified by differences in tension and pressure and by the presence of more or less karatohyalin in their cells, as to suggest that they have had a different origin," says Macleod.

The inner root-sheath is composed of granular polyhedral epithelia, which, in the inner parts, become somewhat elongated, coarsely granular and nucleated. The inner root-sheath covers papilla, forms the bulb or the root of the hair and extends upwards to the neck of the follicle.

"The hair is produced by this sheath alone, by a solid elongation of the epithelia. The inner root-sheath is separated from the outer root-sheath by a thin membrane," says Heitzmann.

Another view of a Dr. Unna is, "Between the inner root-sheath and the main mass of the hair, there is found the matrix from which both the cuticle of the root-sheath and cuticle of the hair are formed."

The cells forming the cuticle of the root-sheath are arranged with their axes on a line with the circumference of the hair, while the cuticle of the hair is composed of cells, which gradually become columnar in shape and lie parallel with the length of the hair.

Hair Bulb or Root

We have already talked about the term *hair bulb or root* of the hair. We know it touches or embraces the papilla and is in turn surrounded by the hair follicle. Hair bulb is composed of three structures; the cuticle (outer skin, epidermis), the cortex (the external part) and the medulla (marrow in various cavities). The thin outer covering or cuticle is a transparent membrane, composed of non-nucleated, imbricated (overlapped) lamellae (thin plate). The cuticle of the hair has an appearance as if made of imbricated scales with elevate eminences, as the root nears the surface. This gives the shaft of the hair a characteristic serrated appearance.

Hair-Shaft

Pluck a hair from your head and hold it against light before your eyes. The plucked place at the root would look like a bulbous white swelling. This white portion of the hair has come out from about two to three millimeters under the skin surface. The place within this skin surface is called root of hair. It produces the actual hair, the body of the hair or shaft. The main *body of the hair or cortical mass* is made of flat, nucleated, delicate but firmly attached fusiform scales that offers a great look to the hair and it appears strong but elastic. Such a quality of the body of hair is further confirmed in the longer hair by central marrow or medulla. Medulla is composed of loosely packed embryonal corpuscles having fatty and pigmented matter. This matter is right from the root of the hair to its end point.

There is a confusion whether these corpuscles have fatty pigmented matters or not? Now the recent studies show that these pigment and fat is air vesicle. The shaft of the hair from scalp or the place of cutaneous exit goes and extends up to its free extremities. This free end of the hair appears healthy and when uncut, it looks like an acuminate point. Such a healthy and pointed shining can be seen on the hairs of normal eyelids. Just examine the eyelid hair of a healthy baby to see this shining at the end of hair of eyelid.

The structure of the hair-shaft is just like that of the hair root (with cuticular, cortical and medullary existence) but without hair-sheaths. In the shaft, the flat like plates of the cuticle are nonmedullated, non-pigmented and overlaid, like that of adherent fish-scales. The cells of the cortex, composing its bulk, are nucleated, pigmented and fusiform. The medulla is absent in the lanugo hairs (the downy hair on the fetus) and is best developed in the strong hair of the eyelashes, moustache and beard.

Hair-papilla

Papillae are spherical or club-shaped originating from the corium and expanding into hair bulbs. The hair papilla is consisting of fibrous and delicate connective tissues, freely supplied with pigmented and non-pigmented connective tissue corpuscles and a variable number of blood vessels. In the opinion of one Dr. Robinson, papillae are nearly twice as long as they are broad and their breadth is in direct proportion to the length of the hairs.

Goose flesh or goose pimples

We have discussed about follicle above. The follicle has a sebaceous (oily, relating to fat) gland and erector pili (hair) muscles. Smooth muscle fibers are attached to the root. Whenever a person gets afraid or alarmed and whenever he or she feels chilly- cold, these pili muscles contract and make the hair stand on end, bunching the skin around the shaft of hair to form an elevated coarse shape *goose pimples.* Small prominences appear on the surface of skin, also called *goose flesh.*

Note :

Readers who know about the structure of skin are accustomed with above medical terms. I have given the meaning of these terms in brackets to make laymen understand the terms.

HAIR AS A PROTECTOR

Hair on our body is a real a gift of God that saves the skin. Hair on the beard and moustaches are natural respirators. You may not believe but hair on the face safeguard our teeth and its frequent shaving may cause bronchitis.

It was Dr. E. H. Ruddock who advocates that keeping beard and moustache is beneficial for the health of throat and lungs. Does this theory make any sense?

We come to hair first. The skin has two main parts, the outer most- the epidermis and under lying layer called dermis. Below the underlying layer is subcutaneous fat. Not going into details of these layers, our concern is that of hair. The cells in the hair follicles form hair and there are two types of hair, the fine and the thick. The fine, downy hair is found over the most of the body except palms, lips, glans penis, inner surface of the prepuce and soles. Thick-pigmented hair is found on scalp, eyebrows, beard and genitals. The thick hair average-growth on the scalp, beard and moustache is 1000 to the square inch. What does it mean? Together the hair forms a sort of shield like a tree over the head and part of face (men).

Body Protection

The hair serve as a shield for head from excessive heat and cold. According to the known values of health, the most delicate part vulnerable to external heat and cold is real of neck, where the collar of the shirt or coat, the hanging cloth of turban, the wrapping of muffler and wearing of a necktie give protection. In women, bunch of tied or loose hanging hair up to shoulders protects the neck or a shield of folded hair in any form or style save them from extremies of climate.

Natural Growth of Nose Hair

Let us come to nose now. Natural growth of hair in the nose is a protector from the diseases of throat, tonsils and lungs. Children who suffer from enlarged tonsils should be trained by the mothers to see that they sleep with their mouths closed. Children sleeping with their mouth open during day or night should be got examined at the earliest and cure of rhinitis or polyps etc., if existing. As a matter of fact, such situations should be taken note of, right from the infancy. We gave no reason to say that hair growth in the nose have no part to play to remove dust particles entering the lungs. If the nasal hair is for the protection of lungs, why not to consider that hair on face also do protection of face and its underneath construction like gums and teeth?

Women and Children without Facial Hair

The question here arises, what about the women and children? If facial hair protects men from stated diseases, how is it that women and children, not having facial hair become victim to these diseases? The probable explanation is that both women and children are not supposed to work outside the homes in hazardous climatic conditions. They are mostly confined to domestic jobs in the house and live in the protected surroundings of home where variation of climate does not take place frequently. Now, when women are out in fields and working outside the homes, they are supposed to be violating the rule of the gender and hence prone to sore throats and bronchitis.

Benefits of Beard and Moustache

And now, a quote from Dr.Ruddock, " The beard and the moustache should be permitted to grow as they afford an excellent protection to the delicate organs of the voice of those in whom it is subjected to undue or irregular exercise. After a public address, the tissues in the vicinity of the throat become relaxed and on leaving the place of assembly and entering the open air, inflammatory action commences, and if repeated, chronic affections of the throat and bronchial tubes are often induced; but the unshorn natural respirator, which our Maker intended to be one of the distinguishing features of the male seed, effectively protects these important parts. The hair planted on the human face by the wisdom and goodness of our Creator, has its uses, and we may add, its beauties. Let the young man, therefore, never become a slave to the false and pernicious fashion which compels him to shave off the beard, as it is found contributory to the health, if not the personal improvement, of those who wear it."

Ruddock recommended growth of beard and moustache not only for prevention of sore throat and hoarseness of voice, but for avoiding bronchitis as well.

According to him, the beard and moustache are a kind of a natural respirator, the shaving off of which is a frequent cause of acute and chronic bronchitis. Can we doubt the wisdom and beneficence of the Creator in giving this ornament to the man, who is so frequently exposed to atmospheric vicissitudes, and withholding it from the woman, who as the keeper at home, requires no such appendage? Hair is an imperfect conductor of both heat and cold and placed round the entrance to the nose and lungs and acts as a blanket, which promotes warmth in cold weather and prevents the dissolving of ice in hot weather. In many instances, the hirsute appendages would protect lawyers, clergymen or other public speakers and singers from the injurious effects of rapid variations of the atmosphere from which professional men so often suffer.

Make a survey yourself

If you, as a practitioner, have been a keen observer, you must have noticed that the patients bearing a beard and moustache (Sikhs in particular) are rarely seen as victims of sore throat, tonsillitis and bronchitis or teeth-gums problems. If you have not made any such observation, do take a note of the patients with a beard in future and you will realize the truth behind this theory of Ruddock. You will find people bearing a beard and moustache and in the range of forty to fifty years of age healthier in all respects when compared with clean shaven persons especially with same age and living in similar environmental entity. In women, you will find the complaints of voice, sore throat more in professionals like teachers or working women indulging in eating out in restaurants.

I have been watching the aspect of beard in many of my patients and in some cases advised bronchitis patients to grow beard / moustache. Keeping a beard and taking homeopathic medicines brought relief sooner than expected. I do not know whether it was the beard keeping or the homeopathic medicine, which acted in favor of the patients but I give some credit to growth of beard too. It is up to you to experiment with your patients. I would suggest that patients having chronic troubles of throat, lungs and toothache be given preference to conduct your experiment.

IDENTIFICATION BY HAIR

Hair is one of the best identification in the body. If a person has committed a crime and there is eyewitness to the crime, the witness would start from the description of hair. Color of hair, long or short hair, crew-cut hair, curly hair, black, brown or gray hair, growth of hair on sides and no hair (bald) can be identified and explained instantly. After all it is hair that crowns the body and it is the first thing to be observed in identifying a person.

Style of hair is another aspect over which the personality and profession of a person can be judged. Those who keep very short hair (men) are generally farmers, army men, technical persons and wrestlers. They are clever, hard working, remain clean and active, make friends with others and mix up easily. Those with long hair are artists, writers, scholars and scientists who have shortage of time for haircuts. They are studious but careless, get irritated easily, reserve type but on provocation, enter into wisely arguments.

In women, the style of hair has different meaning; it is mostly to look different from others. Those with short hair are generally working women and old women who have shortage of time for upkeep of long hair.

Lengthy or short, stylish or flat, the hair have their problems. They are never in stable condition. They are always growing and life ticks every moment within them. Everyday they face winds, storms, dust, sun heat, cold waves and rains. They withstand them all and show symptoms of getting ill, if not cared for in time.

Indian households have certain traditions and traditional diets to maintain the health of hair. The elder ladies of the families know very well that common problems of hair like dandruff and hair loss is the result of poor nutrition, illness, stress, climate and environment and treating the hair in a wrong way such as washing with hot water and use of harsh cosmetics. The common problems of hair are falling, thinning, drying, split ends and breakage. We take birth, live and die. It is the same with hair.

Most of the hair and scalp problems faced by people respond very well with home remedies that are practiced by most of Indian families in many states.

TYPES OF HAIR
Healthy hair

What is the definition of healthy hair? It has been very difficult and even impractical for the best cosmetologist or trichologist to make an assessment or comprehensively define the characteristics of healthy hairs. People assess those hair to be best and healthy which have following qualities:

- Neither oily nor dry.
- Silky and fine.
- Thick, long and dense.
- Shining and glossing.
- Accommodating so that hair can be styled in any fashion.
- Not much of hair loss except in particular seasons.
- Smooth surfaced, remain smooth when wet.
- Tangle little.
- Free of flakes.

In general language (not in medical terms), the hair is formed by cells in the hair follicles and there are *two types* of hair: *fine and thick (coarse) hair.* Very rarely, there is another type called *mixed hair* that are both fine and thick.

Fine

They are downy hairs having a growth all over the body except palms of the hand and soles of the feet. They are silky, soft, shiny and slippery. They dry slowly, if thick and abundant.

Thick

They are coarse, springy, strong or glossy. Thick, pigmented hair have a growth on the scalp, eyebrows, beard and genital areas.

Normal, dry and oily hair

The business community and the manufacturers of cosmetics have devised certain rules of dividing hair, face and skin into three main categories. They have formulated the types of hair in their own rustic way. Most of the cosmetics including creams, lotions, shampoos, hair-dyes and hair colors are available in the market according to this categorization. These three types of hair are *dry hair, oily hair and normal hair.*

Dry hair

Dry hair are those, which have a dry look, appear less elastic and remain dry right from scalp to the end of hair. They have a dry appearance even after application of oil. Dry hair is not the outcome of hereditary effect of genes. There are many reasons behind dry hair. The contributory factors leading to dryness of hair are skin affections, excessive or unsuitable chemical treatment of hair, immoderate heating of hair due to use of hair dryers, excessive setting and styling of hair from the saloons by use of heating appliances, poor diet, and excessive exposure to the sun. During adolescence, the excessive skin flaking found with dandruff due to non-care of hair make hair suitable for yeast infection. Please read 'Hair Care' section of the book.

Oily hair

Oily hair can be distinguished by their oily contents at the scalp whereas the hair ends will appear dry. Oily hair are the outcome of hormonal imbalance, genetic make-up and excessive amount of sebum in the roots of hair. Poor diet, excessive use of cosmetics and adopting harsh hair-care products also lead to oily hair as in the case of dry hair. During adolescence, the sebaceous glands (oil glands) of the scalp are particularly active secreting excess oil. This oil makes the shaft of hair turn oily as a result of which, the hair appears dark, course and lank.

Normal hair

Normal hair are neither dry nor oily and they are really God-gifted, by heredity. They are healthy hair having neither dry nor oily roots and are easily handled in any fashion. To keep the hair in normal condition, one should not resort to factors leading to dry hairs. Basic hair care and nourished diet as observed in such families should be followed instead of deviating to artificial care of hair by use of cosmetics and beauty-appliances. **Wavy, straight and curly** are other types of hair of which we shall know in the chapter 'Care of Hair' in this book.

Color, Curly and Straight Hair

The degree of *straightness or curl, caliber, length and color* depends upon the various structures of body, nationality and races. The hair differs in shape. Straight hair is round in cross section. Curly hair is over shaped. The color of the hair is due to special pigments, varying amount of pigment granules and diffused pigment present in the cortical and medullary portions of the hair and the presence of air, usually in the form of air vesicles. Air vesicles play a vital role in the physiological condition of hair such as gray, white, black, blond, etc.

Hair color depends upon the degree of melanin synthesis, on matrix fibers and spaces between the fibers. The pigment in black and brown hair has *eumelanin* and in light brown hair or red hair, it has *pheomelanin*. Variation of melanin and its compounded melanosomes makes the hair red, brown, black and gray.

Sometimes, there is change of color after prolonged illness and metabolic disorders. This is a different subject and has no relevance in this book. In Indian conditions, we are mostly concerned with black, brown and gray hair and hence are discussed here mainly. Black hair is coarse and rough. In old age, the hair gradually loses its pigments and become gray. The melanogenic activity is reduced as a result of fewer melanocytes and melanosomes along with loss of tyrosinase activity. It is the amount of pigmentation that matters. The degree of pigmentation mostly corresponds to that of other parts of the body-skin. There is variation of growth of hair in races and individuals and also depends upon the state of nutrition caused by rapidly or slowly acting influences on the nerves. If the hair becomes gray before the age 20 to 25, it is due to genetic disorder (familial). Premature gray hair is discussed separately in this book later.

It is the hair *shaft or length that makes the hair curly or straight.* If the hair shaft is cylindrical, hair will be straight. If the hair shaft is oval, the hair will be curly or wavy. We have wooly type hair, as in Africans. If the shaft of hair were flat or kidney-shaped, the hair would look wooly.

HAIRY REGIONS
Hair cover considerable part of the skin. It is absent on the palms of the hands and soles of the feet and certain other parts of the body like dorsum of the distal phalanges of the hands and feet, lips, glans penis and inner surface of the prepuce.

- Every person has a different type of hair on his or her scalp according to the structure of body. They vary in different individuals, nationalities and types.
- There are fine and soft body hair that grow on the trunk

and extremities (fluff).

- There are *long hair* that grow on the scalp. Besides head, long hair grow in the axillae and on the symphisis pubis (genitals) and in case of male also on the face (moustache and beard).
- There are *stiff (bristly)* and short hair that grow on eyebrows.

GROWTH OF HAIR

In terms of growth, hair is classified into three main types: *Anagen, Catagen and Telogen.*

When a new baby is born, he or she has soft, fine and downy hair called *lanugo* that disappears shortly after the birth. Normally hair on the scalp and other parts of body becomes thicker and coarser. In middle age, hair growth can be seen on the ears of men and women develop the same on face at the time of menopause. This is due to change in endocrine pattern.

Anagen Hair *(Period of Active Growth)*

The stage when the growing is in process, the hair is called 'Anagen' hair. Anagen hair keep on growing from two to five years. In Anagen hair, the cells of follicle grow, divide and are keratinized in order to make hair grow. Having keratin means that the base of the hair shaft is moist and soft and the rest of hair shaft above hair bulb is dark pigmented.

Catagen Hair *(Period of Transition or Breakdown and Change)*

When the hair is under transition stage, which is from root to end, the hair is called *'Catagen'* hair. Catagen hair, being transitional, live for about 7 to 15 days. During this transition phase, the growth activity of the hair stops. Growth of hair is not a continuous affair as some people think. Hair growing takes a resting phase during which no growth takes place and the roots of the resting hair become club-shaped. It is this condition that is called *club hairs.*

Telogen Hair *(Resting Stage before Resumption of Growth)*

Catagen hair live for some time and when they are in the state of rest without any change, they are called *'Telogen'* hair. Telogen hair are also called club hair. They are in the state of rest for three to four months before they grow or are pushed from follicle due to growth of another hair or due to some harsh combing / brushing or hard massaging / continuous drying of hair by hot hair-blower or in fight etc. All these are mechanical reasons.

Countless Hair

We cannot count the hair on the head. It varies from person to person. Hair, although abundant in growth, vary considerably in number. *The average growth of hair on the scalp is about 1000 to the square inch, approximately about 120,000 to the entire scalp.* This figure is more, about 140,000 in Blondes and it is less, about 90,000 in redheads (Both Blondes and redheads females or males are not in India but Europe and USA).

Hair growth rate

Hair on the scalp grows on an average of 1.25 cm, say about half an inch, in a month. In cold countries, growth rate is lesser than warm countries. Growth of hair is not a continuous affair as some people think. Every five or six months, hair growing takes a resting phase during which no growth takes place and the roots of the resting hair become club-shaped. Club shaped hair mostly lose their normal pigmentation. Losing normal pigmentation means that the hair become lighter in color. At anyone time, about ten percent of our hair are always in resting phase. It is the club hair that fall when we wash them.

Factors that influence the hair growth

1. **Age :** Growth of hair is fastest from the age of fifteen to late twenties. The hair grow faster and the rate of growth slows down when the hair have grown to its maximum. There is no limit to maximum but some doctors are of the opinion that this limit is three feet and when the hair are over three feet long, the growth rate drops to half the former growth rate.

2. **Nervous and circulatory system :** The hair is affected by the state of the nervous system and circulatory system. This means that hair have a direct relation with functioning of the entire human organism, mind, sentiments, emotions and the body. Any such stimulation in the body by grief, emotions, etc. make impact over the opulence of the nerve and blood supply to the head. If grief or emotions continue for some days, it affects the growth of hair.

3. **Chemicals & Drugs :** Chemical and drug reactions also affect the growth of hair. The coloring of hair and dyeing of hair are virtually exposure to chemical reactions and many persons who dye or color their hair have retarded hair growth or encounter falling of hair.

4. **Heredity :** The heredity/genes actually determine the hair density, growth and color of hair.

5. **Hormones :** Hormonal change is one of the reasons for growth of hair.

Hair Cut or Hair Growth

Every part of the body has some purpose to serve. We cut our hair from scalp and shave our face daily because we do not like its growth to distort our looks (?) and see the obstinacy and compulsion of the body, it brings back the hair we had cut. Is it not sufficient evidence that body contemplates the growth of hair on the place where it suits much to the advantage of skin and the organs beneath it? Actually what we do is we cut the cuticle of hair, which has several parts below i.e. Huxley's layer, Henley's layer, glassy layer medulla, cortical substance, hair bulb, hair papilla, blood vessel and then connective tissues of the cutis, are the parts lying underneath the end of hair, that we cut.

Cutting of hair is a repeated process affecting all the lower parts of the hair in which many changes occur before we see the cuticle come out of skin again. After cutting the end of hair, we cannot rule out the adverse effect on the working efficiency of the blood vessel beneath papilla. The adjoining blood vessels supplying blood to whole of adjoining hair or skin of head and face may not function wholly as per the designed efficiency. In other words, the working efficiency of the hair and the organ beneath is degraded, if not destroyed. There is a saying in our old health books duly approved by our ancestors and saints that cutting of beard could harm gums and teeth. This harm may be in the form of decay or weakness in gums and roots of teeth. Can this be related to malnutrition and inefficiency of blood cells of hair, which are subjected to frequent cuts at its ends? I feel any disturbance caused on the outer body is bound to affect the inner body may be in a long run. It is just like continuous rubbing of the rope drawing bucket of water from the well and resulting in making of a groove on the brick wall of the well. I may be wrong and would like to have a rational correction from your end. I am just correlating theoretical aspects.

Life of Hair

The hair according to above theory has a limited existence and short life. It is shed by the process of separation that takes place about the bulb accompanied by a contraction of the hair- follicle at this point. Once the hair is in its shedding process, the new hair is regenerated from the inner root-sheath about the papilla and it pushes the dead hair lying ahead of it until it is shed or accidentally removed while massaging the scalp or brushing the hair. This means that hair is produced from the epidermis but its production is a process that forms a cornified cylinder, projected from the cutaneous surface and is very analogous to real epidermal cornification. The life of the hair is short but it is a process of regeneration that keeps the healthy person happy when he or she sees the growth of hair returning after a lapse or recess.

Some beliefs

In our Indian families, there is a belief that there is more of hair falling in women when they menstruate. Some people believe that more you cut your hair, more they grow. Some have a belief that shaving has also some effect upon growth rate of hair. All these beliefs have proved to be false.

Data on Growth of Hair

- Trichologists and scientists have studied that average human being has 1,00,000-1,20,000 hair on the scalp.
- A person sheds about one hundred hair everyday on an

average. Ninety percent of these falling hair are 'Anagen' hairs and ten percent of these hair are 'Catagen' or 'Telogen' (Figures are for healthy individuals on an average).

- If one opts not to have a hair cut, the hair would achieve a length of about 106 cm and then would fall.
- When a lady reaches the age range of forty to fifty years, her twenty percent of hair are already fallen.
- With the age reaching forty to fifty years, the hair become dry.
- In a month the hair grow about 12 mm length of hair.
- The speed of hair growing is more during age of fifteen to twenty five or so.
- In summer, the hair growth is more than in winter.
- During sleep, the hair grow more than when awake.

HAIR FALLING

The daily loss of hair from the scalp, on an average, is between fifty to one hundred hair. When the loss of hair exceeds one hundred, this would mean that the production of hair is less or in other words, the hair loss exceeds replacement. This is sign of an approaching baldness. According to one estimate, if the hair loss is plus one hundred every day in autumn and spring, this is not a matter of worry. The weather and the light have impact on hair during this season. Some people, both males and females lose plenty of hair after a cycle of six or seven years. Their hair loss is for about three or four months and then the hair re-grow as normal.

Natural Process of Hair Falling

The wonder of the hair and natural upkeep of the body system suggests that in spite of the handful falling of hair, there is no damage done to the follicles. When the rest of the root is complete after some time or when the root has finished its rest period, normal growth of hair begins again. What an amazing arrangement in our body system? *It means that the body having all normal functions would have falling of those hairs that are in resting phase. This should not be counteracted by induction of medicines. Without any medicines, they would start growing once their resting period is over.* Do we follow it or do we know it? Most of the people do not know it. Had they known it they would not have consulted doctors when they have falling hair.

Chapter 2

Diseases of Hair

Diseases of Hair

Every one is interested to cure his diseases of hair first and then have that glittering shine on his hair that adds charm to the personality. Falling of hair, dandruff, oily or dry hair during particular phases of year are not diseases but disorders because the hair return to their normal state when the phase of certain climates or physical fitness returns. There are many bodily diseases that take away the hair from the scalp. In such cases, the hairs are not diseased but as a result of other diseases, the hair react.

Condition of hair expresses certain diseases as well. So, *condition of hair can be taken as a diagnosis of disease.* Hair is the mirror of health. Lusterless and silky fine hair show tuberculosis. Coarse, thin and dry hair indicate disease of thyroid. There are three main diseases that pinch and add agony to the people. Unruly, bushy hair make a sycotic miasma. Loss of hair in patches and early graying of hair suggest syphilitic diathesis. One streak of gray hair among other black hair express psoric miasma.

The hair-loss, excessive hair-growth and premature gray hair are the three culprits worrying people most. Hair loss and premature gray hair are broad subjects and need elaborations whereas excessive hair growth is a limited topic. Before we discuss about the diseases of hair, it is better to relate to common hair problems in a sum.

These problems are dandruff and flaky scalp, greasy scalp, split ends and head-lice.

DANDRUFF

The common problem of hair now a days is dandruff and almost everyone has experienced this problem during his or her lifetime. Our TV commercials have made dandruff a 'fashion disaster' but there is nothing to worry about. TV commercials also define easy solutions by telling you the brand names of oils or shampoos, which will not only remove your dandruff quickly but win a girl friend too. Every advertisement and products meant for males (shaving creams) have been made female oriented so that male's attraction towards women is never lost sight of and the product is sold out quickly. Dandruff in young boys and girls is a matter of concern in schools or colleges.

What is Dandruff?

It is a disease of the sebaceous glands and there is a secretion of somewhat fatty material that looks on the skin like flakes and scales. Seborrhea of the scalp causes the condition called dandruff. The outermost layer of the skin, epidermis, goes on renewing itself from time to time. The skin sheds dead cells from its surface and are replaced by new cells from underneath. When the amount of production of new cells and this process of shedding is in perfect harmony, there would not be any dandruff. When the production of new cells is less and number of dead cells are more than the new cells, the dead cells or debris of cells get sloughed off in clumps or flakes. *This residue of dead cells is called dandruff.*

It is also common to have little white sand like flakes because this is sloughing off procedure for matured skin cells and debris. People take note of dandruff only when the flakes increase in quantity. Some flakes are dry while others are oily flakes. *It is the dry scales that itch much and it is the oily scales that smell much.* Dandruff is an infectious disease. The personal articles like comb, brush and towel etc. of the person having dandruff should be kept aloof.

Dandruff Infection

This disorder is present in most of people in variable modes. It is an infection where the bacteriological examination states the presence of a *yeast-like organism and staphylococcus,* which in severe cases is found in abundance. This condition is limited to dry scaling of the scalp that may be associated with scaly patches on the forehead and cheeks. Some doctors are of the view that this condition is due to sluggish metabolism, poor diet, hormonal imbalances and infections pertaining to scalp. Recently in USA, some dermatologists have found a different cause in severe cases of dandruff. They hold fungus *Pityrosporum ovale* responsible for severe cases of dandruff. This fungus resides in hair follicles and makes the scalp oily and dandruff greasy. In case, your dandruff is not going even after use of many kinds of dandruff shampoos, it is better to consult a dermatologist who can prescribe some antifungal shampoo or cream or even tablets.

The scales on the scalp may cause some itching and the resultant scratching produces superficial abrasions, which may become infected with the production of impetigo or pustules. If the condition is not treated in time, there is possibility of a slight degree of eczematisation. Under this changed condition, the scalp may develop small rounded pinkish-yellow scaly patches varying in diameter from a quarter of an inch to an inch. Such lesions are called **eczematides.** This mostly occurs on the scalp, forehead and on margin of hair in the form of a 'linear patch having an edge in the form of festoons, a condition called *'corona seborrhoeica'.*

Sometimes dandruff is accompanied by crusts on the scalp and it looks like eczema. The same type of condition exists along the lid margins, on the eyebrows and get scattered over the face in irregular fashion. Dry scaly, rounded, pinkish-yellow eruptions often appear on the pre-sternal and interscapular regions in conjunction with marked *Pityriasis capitis* and they have been termed as *seborrhea corporis,* although no seborrhea is present. Seborrhea corporis is also known as *Flannel rash.* All these terms explained in this paragraph belong to skin. It is not necessary that these skin diseases accompany dandruff. *Pityriasis capitis* is both non-inflammatory and inflammatory and mostly respond well to treatment in all systems of medicines. Salicylic acid and tar are two chemical preparations that bring relief in many skin diseases. Lotions, shampoos, pomades and ointments containing salicylic acid as main constituent are available in the market.

General Causes
- Abrupt change of climate for a person going from cold to hot or hot to cold.
- Wearing tight scarf or tight cap or hat (some doctors or trichologists do not agree with this).
- Not washing the hair in time when they are dirty.
- Tensions and worries.
- Excessive use of hair sprays, gels, colors and dyes.

General symptoms
- White or yellow flakes that come out while scratching or

combing.
- Intense itching of scalp.
- Acne or pimples on forehead.
- Dry flakes on eyebrows or eyelashes.
- White spots on the face.

Treatment

Common man or woman, identifies dandruff when there are flaky dry particles (dead skin) in the hair with an oily sheen. Dandruff arises from oily scalps and not dry scalps. *Most of the people think that dandruff can be removed by washing with medicated shampoo available in the market. To some extent it is true.* It is said that foods that have artificial colors, preservatives of additives should be avoided when dandruff takes place (Please see chapter of food).

The following tips can be followed to get rid of dandruff :

- The best home method is to give a regular treatment to the hair by massaging the scalp with available coconut oil, every night. In the morning, the hair may be washed with shampoo. Massaging mixture of coconut oil, 'Til' oil and 'Amla oil' and washing the hair after one hour of such application removes good lot of dandruff.
- Keeping the hair clean is the best method of treatment in dandruff. And for this, you have to shampoo daily as you comb and brush your hair daily. Selection of a suitable *shampoo is a must in this case.

Note :

*Read more about use and selection of suitable shampoo in **Care of Hair** section of the book.

- Stop using hair styling products on your hair. .
- Stop using cap, turban or 'burqa' (ladies). Wearing such headgears can stimulate the process that is responsible for dandruff.
- In case you have purchased a dandruff shampoo, use it once or twice a week and on other days, use regular shampoo that is not meant for dandruff. This will fetch good results.
- Some experts say that olive oil mixed with rosemary oil when massaged in the scalp instead of coconut oil gives better results. In this case also the hair are to be left overnight after massaging and then washed them in the morning.
- The most common preparation to remove dandruff used to be Glycerin and Eau-de-cologne. People do not use this mixture now. Now most popular method in North India is use of curds mixed with some limejuice. Apply this on the hair and leave them for an hour or so before washing the hairs. It gives good result if no shampoo or soap is used to clear the curds mixture. Application of this mixture, twice or thrice in a week, removes the dandruff.
- Some homeopathic manufacturing companies have brought in some brands of shampoos claiming that they do not have chemicals.
- Brands having certain indigenous herbal plants like 'Reetha', 'Shikakai' and 'Amla', are very useful.
- There are soaps that claim containing 'Triffla' with 'Shikakai'. To some people these soaps (marketed in pink and black colors) have been found useful (Trade-names of soaps not given for obvious reasons).
- It is said that gentle massaging of table salt on the scalp and leaving the same for fifteen minutes and then washing removes dandruff.

- Before washing the hair, massage some vinegar on the scalp and leave it for one hour. Wash the hair after that. Repeat this twice or thrice in a week.
- It is also the frequency of washing the hair that becomes a tool for removing the dandruff. In winter, people wash their hair only once a week thus allowing dust to accumulate in the hairs. This aggravates the condition.
- Two tablespoonful of malt vinegar should be added in a glass having 250 ml of water. Shampoo your hair and then rinse the hair with this solution. Dry the hair in natural way.
- Avoid eating fried food, nuts, chocolates and animal fat.
- Take milk and its products, green vegetables, fish, chicken and products that contain Vitamin A, E and B complex.
- Two tablespoonfuls of 'methi' seeds should be soaked in water overnight. Next morning, grind the seeds and make a paste. Apply this paste on the hair and leave them for an hour. Rinse the hair with fresh water using a good herbal shampoo.
- Grind four teaspoon of 'Khas-khas' in some milk and apply on the roots of hair. Let it remain on the hair for half an hour and then wash the hair with shampoo. Do this twice a week.
- In a cup of curd, mix some salt and shake it with little water. Rub the mixture in the hair and then wash the hair after half an hour.
- Take four teaspoon of 'Besan' and make a paste of it in water. Apply this and let it remain for about fifteen minutes. Wash the hair with shampoo.

Quick Removal of Dandruff

- Warm two teaspoonful of castor oil (quantity according to length of hair). Massage this lukewarm oil into hair twice or thrice a week at night. Leave the oil overnight and wash your hair in the morning. Continue this procedure for two weeks and you will find dandruff gone.

• Dilute some cider vinegar in water and add some lavender oil. Massage this oil in the hair every night. Wash your hair in the morning. Do it for seven days and you will find dandruff gone.

Treatment of Flaky Scalp

If you are using very harsh shampoos, which have hard chemicals, there is possibility that the scalp may develop flakes and these should be avoided. Of course, poor diet, stress and lack of sebum also imbalance the hair texture and produce flakes. Moisture rich shampoo and some good conditioner generally removes the flakes.

Treatment of Greasy Scalp/oily hair

People having a greasy scalp should not worry much about it. If they do not apply the oil over the hair regularly, they will loose the hair. The best is to adopt the homeopathic method, 'Like cures like'. Add oil to the greasy scalp. Since the scalp itself is producing more of oil, the presence of oil on the scalp would stop production of oil from within. The imbalance will thus be overruled. If you are washing the hair twice a week (women), apply oil, massage it into scalp and leave it for at least one hour before washing it with shampoo. If you are a male, do it five times a week.

Some doctors and trichologists do not agree with this theory and say that frequent washing and less of oil application removes the condition of greasy hair. It is better to consult a cosmetic clinic when you do not find any relief in adopting above methods because you will need conditioners to rectify the greasy scalp.

An US study states that *'Baby shampoo'* available in the market is good for removing excessive oil from the hair. This shampoo is mild due to its alkaline nature but it is a great degreasing agent. If this suits, go on using this shampoo otherwise purchase some shampoo meant for oily scalp have drying agents like zinc sulphide etc.

If you wash your hair with shampoo twice a day, it will remove the oily nature of hair but this may not be possible in India where people are very busy in their jobs and professions.

A *check up of hormones* is also useful although oily scalp has nothing to do with genes. If the scalp had been dry earlier and it has turned oily after use of some medicines or birth control pills then stop taking of pills for some time and check the result.

Treatment of Split Ends

Hair split ends is the condition of hair mostly known to women. Some of the hair bunches at the ends form splitting. Split is lengthwise division of the hair. In this condition, the cuticle of hair gets damaged and the fiber of the cortex becomes disentangled (unraveled).

This condition happens due to use of harsh soaps, shampoos and hard chemicals. To rectify the hair split ends, there is no treatment. *It is better to cut the split ends of the hairs and for this, you have to go to the hairdresser or a beauty saloon.* The hairdressers take small sections of hair-strands and twist them and scissor up and down the hair shaft to cut any stray ends which appear raising above the whole level of hair. It is an art to cut the split end hair and one should not try it at home.

Treatment of dandruff by homeopathy, shall be discussed later in this book.

MATTED HAIR (PLICA)

I have seen children in villages having this disease of matted hair and you must have seen roaming seers and saints having matted hair. 'Jatta ban jana' is the Hindi term for matted hair. In seers and saints, it is done deliberately and proper care is taken that no infection takes place on the scalp. City people do not have this disease, which relates more to cleanliness than skin. Plica is a condition in which hair is matted together due to filth and dust. Not only the dust is allowed to accumulate but also it is not cleaned / combed and it remains there on the head for some period. The result is inflammation of scalp and matted hair.

Treatment

The treatment is simple. Cut short the hair nearly up to the skin and do not shave the head clean. Keep the hair clean and the remaining matted hair near the scalp should be tangled with comb and brush dipped in warm water. Homeopathic medicines can be given for this disease according to symptoms. Borax veneta, Acidum fluoricum, Lycopodium clavatum and Sarsaparilla are the medicines to be thought over. Homeopath should be consulted for this.

BARBER'S ITCH

Barber's itch is a term well known to people and they relate it to some inflammation or eruption on the beard or scalp after a visit to a barber's shop. It is an inflammatory disease of the hair follicles of the beard and moustache because of microbial infection. There is appearance of nodules, pustules or papules. The lesion can be in limited area or scattered on a big area or grouped in one area. Once it appears, there may be gradual increase of the infection from one follicle to the other. Initially when the infection starts, the hair can not be pulled without pain but as the suppuration takes place and is active, the hair can be easily plucked without any pain. In some cases, the pustular secretion comes up in small crusts and in severe cases, the crusts is more and may exhibit a weeping surface. The infection does not spread on non-hairy parts of the body. There may be burning, itching and some sort of discomfort felt but all symptoms are mild without any troublesome indications. The condition is generally limited to beard. The patients are males between the ages of 20 years to 50 years. The disease is transmissible by contagion from the use of razor or blade previously applied for shaving other person affected with infection.

Treatment

The factor that brings in this disease has to be removed and is of primary consideration. As stated above, it is better not to get the shaving done from barber shop and if it is unavoidable, see that the barber changes the blade or boils the razor in water before use. The towel used should be fresh and washed. After the shave, it is better to wash the face with water and apply alum stone or some antiparasitic / antiseptic ointment. Hot borax water is also good for washing the face. When the beard is already having the infection, one should shave at home with utmost care although it may be little painful. The homeopath uses following medicines and the treatment should be under his guidance.

Cicuta virosa, Lachesis mutus, Graphites, Lycopodium

clavatum, Rhus toxicodendron, Petroleum, Tellurium metallicum and Sulphur.

HEAD LICE
(Lice Infestation-Pediculosis or Pediculus Humanus)
('Joo-en' in Hindi)
The common cause of lice infestation in the hair is supposed
to be carelessness in cleaning of the scalp and hair. Most of
us believe in this theory of clean scalp but the fact is that
presence of lice in the human hair is not because of poor
hygienic conditions or dirty hair. According to a latest study by
U.S.A. researchers, the lice prefer to lay its eggs on clean hair
and scalp. Normally long hair is more infested with lice.

The louse is a parasitic insect that gets transmitted by head
to head contact of people, sharing hair-brushes and combs,
sharing and lending hats, soaps and towels to others. The
children acquire the lice from their classmates, youngsters get
them from public conveyance, sleeping on other's beds and
using other's clothing. Those who get infection are children and
people who work with them, the teachers.

The louse is an insect without wings although people think
that it flies from one head to the other. It is smaller than a match
stick-head and gray in color. It turns to brownish gray after
sucking blood from the skin. It moves from one head to the
other and lays eggs on the hair with cement like secretion so
that the eggs stick on the hair shaft. It lays its eggs, called 'nits'
(Leekhen' in Hindi) along the base of the hair shaft, close to the
scalp. Their eggs hatch within eight or nine days after being
laid. They look white like dandruff and they remain farther
from the scalp than the lice themselves.

Louse has six claw-like legs (feet) that help it cling firmly
to the hair-shaft. It has two trunk-like whiskers that help it to

suck blood. It feeds itself by drawing blood from the scalp. The scalp infestation by the lice makes the scalp itch and later it causes bacterial infection. The bite of lice irritates the skin and children cannot resist itching. This disturbs their sleep also.

Lice are also responsible in spreading fevers like relapsing fever, typhus fever and trench fever. Most of the factors, which conduce to the spread of typhus fever and relapsing fever, operate by their influence on the parasites by which the disease is conveyed. The lice pass directly from the sick to the healthy or by means of garments, bedclothes and mattresses, which have been in contact with those infected. Trench fever was first reported in First World War. It is a blood infection communicable from man to man by means of the louse. This fever created lot of problems in the World War-I. Let us not go into details of this fever or other fevers. It was because of this infection that possibly army framed a rule to go in for crew-cut hairstyle (short hair) for soldiers so that lice cannot breed there smoothly.

The only precaution is that in all types of fevers, which last long, one must see that lice are eradicated.

Treatment

Many beauty parlors and experts claim that the lice infestation can be cleared with a single application of medicines. Application of 25 percent of benzyl benzoate emulsion or one percent of gamma-benzene hex a chloride or two percent of DDT emulsion mostly remove the lice infestation. There are branded lotions available in the market with which lice infestation is removed. It is up to the user to think whether such harsh insecticides treatment is necessary or not.

People do not prefer above mentioned treatment if you care for your skin and hair. *Natural methods to eradicate the problems of lice infestation are far better and popular even in advance countries.*

Adopt following procedure to eradicate lice from the head of your child:

- Keep separate towel, oil and soap for the child, away from the rest of belongings of the family.
- Wash the hair and apply a conditioner that has silicon as base (available in the market).
- Use a comb that has teeth with wide placement so that the entanglement of hair is eased first.
- In the second stage now, comb the hair with a lice-comb (available in the market). This comb has very fine toothed-placement to remove the lice after each stroke. Part the hair in section so that after each stroke, you can see the lice in the comb. Rinse the comb so that lice are removed. Turn by turn; make sections of hair and go on removing the lice by rinsing each time.
- Repeat this wet-comb method every other day so that all the lice are removed.
- All the lice will be caught in this method and they would not be able to hatch.
- Combing the hair with lice-comb and after every stroke, dipping the comb in hot mug of warm water also catches the lice. This can be done every day.
- You cannot remove eggs of lice (nits) with this comb method because they stick on the hair shaft.
- Nits can be removed with the help of fingernails. This is a method prevalent in Indian homes and is quite useful.
- Apply **olive oil** generously on the scalp and leave it overnight. Wash the head next morning with some good shampoo. Repeat this washing every third day for about three weeks.
- Use of **carbolic soap** also helps in killing lice but one

should watch if some eruptions come up on the scalp.

- **If possible, the long hair may be cut short.** This is one of the best methods to remove lice early. The lice cannot maintain a mechanical hold over the hair and cannot establish themselves. In long hair, lice have no difficulty of optimum temperature that insects require to produce eggs. In increased temperature, lice are comfortable. Cutting the hair short means affecting their life with decreased temperature.

- The leaf of beet be boiled in water and then allow it cool down. Now wash hair with this water and you will find head- lice dead after few applications for some days.

Homeopathic Treatment

- Take 10 ml each of *Sabadilla-Q, Ocimum-Q* and *Azadirachta-Q* and mix them. Apply this as a lotion on the hair and leave it for about two hours and then wash the hair. Repeat this two to three times in a week.

- If this does not work, Take 30 ml of *Staphysagria-Q* and mix it with 120 ml of water. Apply this on the head in the same above manner and wash. Along with this external treatment, give the child *Staphysagria-30* three times daily internally for one week and check the results.

- One weekly dose of *Psorinum 200* and daily use of *Carbolicum acidum 30,* three times a day for one week works to eradicate lice. With this medication, use the wet comb method to remove the lice externally.

Note :

It is better to use above medicines under the guidance of homeopath.

- *Vinca minor 30* may be taken three times a day for one week if the hair are matted and have lice in them.
- *Staphysagria 30* may be taken three times a day for one week, if the lice are in pubic hair also. For local application, this medicine in mother tincture is useful. 1 Dm of *Staphisagria-Q* and 1 oz of coconut oil should be mixed and mixture applied daily for a number of days.

Dr. E.P. Anshutz was a renowned homeopath of Philadelphia and he wrote a book "Therapeutics By-ways". In this book, he gives an interesting description on lice. He says, "Some children seem to attract lice like molasses does flies. Von Villars reported such a case and cured it with Staphysagria 30th, internally. Seems absurd, but so it was reported. The mother told him in answer to his first rough, "Why don't you keep the child cleaner?" that she did, but no matter how often she washed and combed it the lice would soon appear. Well, with unbelief, he gave Staphysagria 30 and, after one washing, the lice never appeared again. So reported in an old German Medical Journal."

HYPERTRICHOSIS AND HIRSUTISM
(Hair Growth On Unwanted Places)
Both **hypertrichosis** and **hirsutism** are the terms applied to an excessive growth of hair. If you happen to visit a crowded swimming pool or had been to 'Har-ki-pauri' at Haridwar, you must have noted many persons having strong hair growth on their neck, back, chest, elbows, ears and so on. Excessive growth of hair at unwanted sites of the body is a condition called hypertrichosis. It is usually confined to those cases in which a growth of stout hair occur in sites

usually covered with lanugos hair, such as the face in women.

The amazing part of this disease is that people do not bother to consult a doctor and take it as a normal gift from God. As a matter of fact, such persons do not show their concern about the condition outwardly but develop a sort of depression, causing a serious effect on their mental condition. Hypertrichosis can be treated and it should receive consideration. Dermal tumors and sites of melanocytic nevi also have this growth of hair on them. Strong hair are present in pigmented moles and they are seldom larger than several square centimeters. Very occasionally, a male seeks advice regarding hypertrichosis on the trunk. Hair on the trunk are mostly seen in males and they do not consider it as any abnormality.

The most depressed condition of excessive hair growth is found in women and this is also called **'Hirsutism'** although hypertrichosis is considered a broad and right word. The chin and cheeks are the areas usually affected and the disorder varies from a few strong hair on each side of the chin to profuse growth affecting the area near upper lips, cheeks, chin and neck. In some cases, the growth is also on central chest, breasts, lower abdomen and groins. In Punjab and Haryana, elderly ladies having excessive growth of hair on face are typed as women with masculine quality of courage. In villages, they are respected. Sometimes the growth of hair on the face is so much that people call the woman as 'bearded woman'. It is mostly congenital and has a bearing with certain races too.

Variation in races has to be considered for hirsutism. Indian women have very little hirsutism if compared to women of other countries. Russian women have hirsutism in abundance but they do not bother much about it. Similarly, women of South European and Middle Eastern countries have hirsutism more than their Indian counterpart.

F-5

Causes

1. **Heredity :** In most of the cases, hypertrichosis is congenital. In some cases, it is reported that the mother took drugs during pregnancy resulting in hypertrichosis and other associated features like wide and large, lips and mouth with short neck. Congenital syphilis is also one of the reasons for this disease. The hair is often shed extensively but on the other hand, syphilitic infants may grow an abundant crop of hair, which has been called the 'syphilitic mop' though it occurs in other diseases.

2. **Virilism:** It is seen that in some cases, hirsutism is associated with signs of virilization (appearance of secondary male characteristics in the female) that has balding temples, deepening of voice, acne and clitoral hypertrophy.

3. **Drugs & Disease :** In the cases where hypertrichosis is acquired, it may be a result of lipoatrophic diabetes and other syndromes like Lange, Hurler, and Morogu etc. Use of some typical steroids also becomes cause of hypertrichosis. Use of androgens and certain high progesterone birth control pills (though not so common) also cause hirsutism. Use of drugs like corticosteroids, phenytoin, diazoxide and minoxidil are also reported to produce hirsutism. These can produce abundant of hair-growth on any part of the body besides face. In cases, where some limbs of the body have grown dispropor-tionate to the rest of body (a condition called 'Acromegaly'), the growth of hair may be more and they become coarse also.

4. **Menopause & Endocrines :** Hypertrichosis or hirsutism can develop at any age, if it is not by birth. Many women get excessive hair growth on their face when they are

approaching menopause. It is not with all the women. In most of the cases, it is not possible to find out single apparent cause for the growth of excessive hair. Some endocrine disorder is equally responsible for this extraordinary 'shock' for women.

5. **Cosmetics :** I am not very sure about Indian women but it has been seen that women in USA and other developed countries are extra aware about their looks. Reaching old age is a natural biological phenomenon but these women try to deceive the age and take extra precautions, when they grow old. They use Vaseline, cold creams and greasy applications repeatedly as if to cover their wrinkles or avoid wrinkles. Such greasy cosmetics are supposed to favor extra hair-growth. Some doctors do not agree with this cause because such creams are used widely and everyone does not get hirsutism. Greasy skin does not mean development of hirsutism it is not a predisposing factor.

6. **Hormones :** Some doctors opined that hormonal changes in the body make a difference. Hirsutism may be due to excessive secretion of androgens from either the ovary of the adrenal gland or from excessive stimulation by pituitary tumors. The secretions in excess may be due to functional excesses or from neoplastic processes.

Homeopathic Treatment

It is observed that not much can be done with the help of homeopathy in this disease. Many homeopaths claim that they have cured cases of hirsutism but my practical experience of thirty five years show that homeopathy takes a very long course of time to stop the excessive growth of hair. The patients do not have much of patience to see the results of homeopathic medicines and hence I could not confirm even a single case, where I had cured any lady of this problem. The patients leave the treatment and are probably lured by easy solution of mechanical removal of hair by laser and other methods. If someone is interested in homeopathy, following medicines can be tried.

— *Thuja occidentalis 1M* – one dose every month for about 6 months to see the results. Failing this, *Oleum jecoris aselli* may be started.

— *Oleum jecoris aselli 3x* – Two doses daily for twenty days and then no medicine for ten days. Again repeat the medicine for twenty days with gap of ten days. Repeat this cycle for six months.

— **Dr. R.B. Bishambar Das** suggests that *Oleum jecoris aselli* may be given in 30 potency in summer and in 3x potency in winter thrice daily along with *Thuja occidentalis* 1M. *Oleum jecoris aselli* is not to be given two days before or after giving *Thuja occidentalis.*

Besides this, he suggests that mechanical method should be adopted for removal of facial hair. He advises that yellow sulphate of arsenic and quick lime in equal parts be mixed in hot water to make a paste. This paste be applied on the face and allow it to dry. No hair will show there for weeks.

— **Dr. J. N. Shinghal** suggests that *Thuja occidentalis* 200 should be given every month and *Oleum jecoris aselli* 3x be given thrice daily except on the day when *Thuja occidentalis* is taken.

— **Dr. T. P. Chatterjee** says that *Thuja occidentalis* 200 should be given weekly and Oleum jecoris aselli 3x be given twice daily excepting the day on which Thuja accidentalis is taken till the growth stops. Further for growth of excessive hair on child's face, Calc., Nat-m., Ol-j., Psor. and Sulph. should be tried according to other symptoms of the body. Actually, **Kent** suggests the same for child's facial hair growth.

— According to **Kent's** repertory, for hair on unusual parts, there are two medicines indicated, Med. and Thuj. The same is for treatment of hairy parts.

Therapeutics

Hair all over the body: Aru., Thyr., Med.

Hair on odd parts: Thuj., Thyr., Lyc.

Hair on children faces: Nat- m., Calc., Psor., Ol- Jec 3x.

Treatment : Conventional and Mechanical

Very occasionally, you will find a male seeking advice regarding hirsutism on the trunk and back. In other cases, take the instance of moles on the body having streaks of hair in them. Strong hairs are found in pigmented moles and these moles are large in some cases but still these are not bothered about because these are seldom larger than a few square centimeters. Also, a tuft of well-developed long hair is seen arising from the skin overlying a spina bifida (a congenital defect in which the vertebral neural arches fail to close) in some cases but the males do not bother about these petty disorder.

Women are very much conscious about their looks and excessive hair growth on unwanted places. The best way to remove hair from face is to get them removed. There are many methods available for removal of hair. Both cosmetics and mechanical methods are cheapest. Shaving is the best method but women and girls do not like it due to social restrictions. Some women use a piece of soaped pumice stone to scrub away the hair instead of using a razor. This takes time and is again considered unsocial in the present era when hair- removing creams are available in plenty. There are waxes (epilatory) and chemical depilatories for this purpose.

1. **Depilatory remedies :** The *depilatory remedies are not injurious or costly. Every brand of hair removing cream, wax or soap has its secret formula. But in all these preparations, the sulphides of barium and calcium are the ingredients commonly used. Sulphides of barium is mixed with equal parts of oxide of zinc and starch to make a thick cream in water. This cream is spread on the hair required for removal and left there to dry up for ten minutes. After ten minutes, the area is washed and the dissolved hair come out with it. Most of the products carry instruction-manuals with the pack of cream and the instructions should be followed to remove the hair. If the cream is prepared with sulphide of calcium, it destroys the hair rather farther down the follicle and produces inflammation. Sulphide of barium does not produce inflammation as much as sulphide of calcium. This inflammation is mostly temporary but later there are chances that some kind of eczema can spurt out on the skin in some cases.

2. **Epilating waxes :** Most of ·women prefer epilating waxes. Epilating waxes are made of beeswax and rosin. Wax removes the hair temporarily. Epilatory waxes have advantages over depilatory waxes because their use is not attended with the risk of inflammation, eczema or chemical burns. However a patch test is needed before

Note :

* Both the terms depilatory and epilatory mean removal of hair. The constituents in both make them different.

use of epilating waxes/hair remover cream. On the area of application, some cream is applied and after ten minutes, it is wiped off. Wait for twenty-four hours and then check the area. If there is no inflammation or rashes on the applied area, the cream can be used safely. The cream is spread generously and evenly over the skin from which the hair is required to be removed. No rubbing of cream is needed. The application should be left for about ten minutes and then wiped off gently with damp cloth or cotton wool. Next, the area is washed with lukewarm water and wiped with soft towel. No soap is applied for washing. In this process, the incorporated hair are pulled out smoothly. Whole procedure is painless. Epilating waxes are available under branded names like hair remover creams. Key-ingredients in hair remover cream are thioglyocollic acid, calcium hydroxide and fragrance.

3. **Bleaching :** Bleaching the hair with equal parts of hydrogen peroxide with liquid ammonia makes them less conspicuous and has a beneficial corrosive action on the finer hair. It makes the hair less dark and thus less noticeable. If some oiliness is felt after bleaching, it can be treated by the use of spirituous degreasing lotions. Bleaching should not be done at home. This facility is available in beauty parlors.

4. **Hormones :** Some women resort to endocrine therapy (hormonal) including use of the newer ovarian preparations. This is mostly found disappointing.

   There is a notion that removal of hair by plucking, shaving or waxing brings more of hair growth in the area. This has been proved false.

5. **Electrolysis :** The oldest method adopted by women is 'electrolysis'. It consists in passing a current of about 1

milliampere for a quarter to half a minute into the hair bulb by means of a fine needle attached to the negative pole of a galvanic battery. The hair thus loosens and can be removed. It is very essential that the hair should not to be removed too close to one another at the same sitting. If it is done in one sitting, there may be troublesome scaring left. The experts working in beauty parlors should take care of it.

    (i) Pulsed light treatment : A still modified method of electrolysis is pulsed light treatment that takes about five to six sittings for removal of hair. This is painless and there are no marks left on the skin.

6. **Diathermy coagulation :** It is considered most satisfactory method of treatment of hypertrichosis of moderate degree on the face or removal of hair from moles. In this method, the experts use a very fine needle attached to minimal coagulation current. This needle is inserted into the hair follicle and down to the air root, which is then coagulated. Diathermy coagulation is supposed to be much better than electrolysis because it is easier for the patient and speedy in removing more of hairs in one sitting. The only drawback of this method is that if the operator or the professional is not well skilled, the risk of scarring is greater than electrolysis.

7. **Light-sheer diode laser :** With the advance of science, the beauty experts have introduced permanent 'excess body hair removal method' called 'Light sheer diode laser' method. This method claims that no further growth of unwanted hair take place. I am not very impressed about this statement calling 'permanent removal' and it sounds like 'permanent' dyes available in the market. One thing is certain that new

methods are supposed to be better than the previous methods. In electrolysis and diathermy coagulation, the results appear disappointing and repetition is needed after some period. *Quite a number of hair reappear and the procedure has to be repeated.* It is, therefore, made clear to the patient that hair removal is not permanent and there will be more of time and sittings needed.

One thing is sure that by removal of unwanted hair, the patient gets mental satisfaction and time spent is thus not taken seriously. Now a day, when the women visit beauty parlors more frequently for petty jobs like threading, bleaching, face cleaning, facial, manicure, pedicure, massages, full leg waxing, full arm and under arm waxing or hair cuts, they can devote some of the time for facial hair removal along with other schedule tasks. This is applicable for urban folks who are much conscious about their looks and visit beauty parlors frequently. For village belle, there is no need for hair removal. Their natural beauty with sparkling health covers all the scars, facial hair or dark spots.

FALLING OF HAIR / HAIR LOSS (ALOPECIA)

There is a piece of advice in 'Charka Samhita' (Sutra sathanam, 5th Chapter, shaloka 81-82) on care of hair. It reads as follows in Sanskrit:

'Nityam snehadaram shirsa shira sholam na jayte
Na kahalitayam na palitiyam na kasha parpatanti cha'

It means that one should apply oil on the hair daily, regularly and massage them so that the hair are lubricated (not dry). This way, there is no headache, the hair do not get weak, they do not fall and they do not get gray prematurely.

This advice should not be forgotten. The hair fall problem is due to dryness in the body, malnutrition, keeping the hair wet for a long time, dandruff, late night sleep, tensions, worries and not applying oil as per the fashion of the day.

Hair loss before the age of thirty to thirty-five years is supposed to be awkward and people resort to many methods for bringing back the lost hair. If you happen to see pictures of characters shown in various religious and historical books, you will find many persons above the age of forty having bald and shaven heads. In ancient history of India, Hindu scholars and priests are shown shaven-headed with a strand of hair (choti) falling behind. 'Chanakya', the wise minister of 'Chanderagupta' was one of those characters. The reason behind such ritual of keeping 'choti' was made essential by priests because they had probably lost their hair. In young age they held long hair falling over their backs. Once the hair started falling due to age factor, they resorted to 'priest' fashion. If you have seen the old film, 'Samson and Delilah', (Translated film 'Aurat' in Hindi, where part of Samson was played by actor Prem Nath), you will remember that Samson had all his power in hair. He could even lift an elephant. When his hair were shaved, his power got lost. It is a fiction but the writer of the era exhibited a general notion of the times that hair is a symbol of strength.

In the Middle East, Egypt, we have known about preserving dead bodies in the ancient times. These are called 'Pharaoh' or 'mummy'. The mummy invariably wears a wig. Probably, hair loss in countries like Egypt, Rome and Greece was more in the olden days and hence the inhabitants preferred to wear wigs to protect themselves from heat and sun. Even after death of a person, when mummy of the body was prepared, wig was not forgotten.

If hair was considered so important, how is it that olden

days doctors or 'Hakims' did not find any remedy for growth of hair? As a matter of fact, hair loss has been a long-standing problem to which no cure has been found. The ancient doctors tried hard to get a remedy but failed. Many types of lotions, oils and soaps were invented but without any benefit.

In this world of high technology and advance medical knowledge, *there is no medicine or lotion by which fallen hair can be grown or bald man or women get back their full growth of hair.* Fake and bogus hair treatment to cure baldness has always been popular not only in India but in other advance countries too. Knowing that the manufacturer's claim is tricky and bogus, people fall to the lure of advertisements and spend money but do not get the desired results. The persons who go bald are so curious and intent to grow hair that they would do anything suggested. *The amazing part of this story of hair loss is that medical scientists, doctors and beauty experts have different opinions about this so-called tragedy of youth. Every one has different explanation.* There is, of course, no denial that falling of hair has a different treat for different persons, different ages and different rate of falling of hair. There is a natural balance between the rate of falling and rate of growing of new hair but this is not applicable to all.

Once the falling of hair starts, people do not want to wait and check the causes. They consult the doctors even if the cause of falling is due to climatic changes. *They desire immediate treatment.* One should not expect quick results without making any remedial measures and taking professional help. It takes time for hair to grow. The hair might have been growing after falling but there is lack of patience to wait and watch. The medicines and oils or applicants are used as if these agents would speed up growing.

If you have full crop of hair crowning the head, you are lucky and people looking at you would appreciate this.

Having good growth of hair in spite of several pressures of speedy and competitive life at domestic and work level is a matter of pride. Youth today is very conscious about looks and especially hair. An onset of slight falling of hairs makes them anxious. Falling of hair or hair loss is a typical phenomenon. See the irony of the situation, people still believe in the 'advertising hype' exhibited in TV and newspaper media. The hair treatment business for preventing hair loss, turning gray hair to black and removing dandruff is to the tune of several crores of rupees. The various hair product industries have huge advertising budget so that people are carried away by the colorful advertisements. These companies take the help of sex appeal and show how women are attracted to men once they return to good hair growth. Hair has been continuing to be sign of youth and vigor. When the youth fails to restore his or her hair in spite of using the prescribed brands of medicines, he or she turns to wearing wigs, the sale of which is considerably more in USA, UK and other European countries. In India, it is not common to wear wigs. Newspapers and magazines are full of advertisements for costly hair growth tablets and applicants and people in India are lured easily for these products, which are not useful enough to restore what is lost. Papers in UK are full of such advertisements with addresses of hair clinics that sell worthless scalp massages, hair growing lotions and tablets. Even intelligent men and women fall pray to this sort of claims. It is because they would do anything to look younger by restoration of hair on their heads.

Let us form an opinion now about hair falling and baldness. We shall be using term **'Alopecia'** henceforth. Alopecia is loss of hair, partial or general, varying from a mere thinning to complete baldness. The degree of falling may be such that it starts from thinning of hair and then complete baldness. We have already discussed that some hair fall everyday due to some physiological reasons. The normal life of a hair on the scalp is about 3-4 years after which it is shed and is then replaced by the new cells forming from the germinal matrix. Falling of hair may be due to structural and functional disorder in the follicle or to a change in the hair itself. It is mostly noted that *falling of hair occurs in the morning*. There is no answer to this phenomenon. I have personally enquired from some reputed cosmetologists, dermatologists and trichologists but no one could give suitable explanation. I came to know about a new phenomenon that *longer hair have decreased rate of hair falling*. It needs verification.

Hair Loss : Disease ?

Average hair loss is about thirty to one hundred a day. This is normal. One should test the actual loss so that they know whether they suffer from alopecia. Comb the hair for four days in the morning i.e. a day before washing the hair, a day on the washing of hair and two consecutive days after washing the hair. Count the number of hair fallen each day and add them. If the average comes to 100 hair per day, its not hair falling disease.

Types of Alopecia

Alopecia is mainly of two varieties, *temporary and permanent* and to conclude this, one has to examine them in respect of time taken to reach such baldness. Time scale can be enormously different in each case. People suffering from alopecia have different views about themselves. Some take it granted that it is due to hereditary effect and keep quite after using some of the products available in the market. They assert themselves that it is a matter of natural personality and fate. The period of hair loss is between the twenties and fifties of the age.

In general, a person on an average loses 50 to 100 hair a day and mostly all of it grows back. This is temporary alopecia, if you choose to call it falling of hair.

Permanent alopecia is the main alopecia we have been discussing and we shall be learning more about it later in this book.

Temporary alopecia

The general perception is that temporary hair loss is on account of poor nutrition, illness, stress, incorrect or harsh treatment of hair, side effects of some medications, childbirth and hormonal imbalance. Hair loss is associated with two phases: the temporary condition or from long term condition i.e., age-related changes. Our respected old men and women at homes have unique treasure of advice based on 'hear and say' belief learnt from their elders. *According to them, hair loss is mainly due to tension and worries.*

Here is a modern explanation to what our elders say. With worries, the skin of scalp goes under tension. It contracts and tightens the scalp. This prevents sufficient nutrient-rich blood from reaching the hair follicles and the hair roots get starved, resulting in shrinkage and then ultimately falling of hair prematurely.

- Temporary alopecia is the one that is either self induced or has been habituated. For example, some people have the habit of plucking hair from scalp and eyelashes and even nasal hair. This neurotic practice is found mostly in children. This is a temporary habit and once it is checked, the alopecia is gone.

- The other temporary alopecia is due to **compulsive pressure.** The infants are generally having it. They develop thinning of hair at the occipital area due to their continuous lying on their backs. In adults also, it is developed in persons who are in coma, having illness or under prolonged bed rest, say induction of general anaesthesia etc. Their occipital area goes under constant pressure due to above conditions and thus a temporary alopecia is created.

- The next temporary alopecia is **pulling or traction alopecia.** It occurs when the hair are under constant pull for hours everyday. If the hair are tightly braided or dressed in a ponytail fashion, pulled frequently to straighten the hair or twisting the hair with fingers to make a knot and tie with rubber band or rolling curlers too tightly, there is likelihood of temporary alopecia. Tight plaiting may also bring in loss of hair at the sides of the base of plait. Tightening the hair and attaching hairpieces or clips also bring in the same result. In all such cases, it has to be observed that the hair loss site gets the growth after the tightening habit is left. If the hair do not grow from the area, traction alopecia may turn to permanent hair loss.

- Use of hot air and hot comb to straighten the hair also bring in temporary alopecia.

As a matter of fact, *it is very difficult to mark a line of division between temporary and permanent hair loss* because no one knows whether the hair are returning to normal growth or not after a temporary falling after sickness, pregnancy and leaving all the above mentioned rituals.

Male Type Alopecia (Androgenic)

Alopecia or loss of hair in males differs from the alopecia of females. It is known as *male pattern baldness.* It is very common type of baldness and most of men suffer from it. Degree of severity varies from trivial to extreme. Male pattern baldness is on account of disorder of male hormones, which are collectively known *as androgens.* The hormone connected with male pattern hair loss is *testosterone.* Hormones are chemical messengers produced by the body that stimulates activity by organs or tissues elsewhere in the body. If a man has inherited the genes responsible for hair loss, a little of this testosterone is made by some of the hair roots into a derivative named as *dihydrotestosterone.* This dihydrotestosterone is mostly responsible for male pattern hair loss.

In males, alopecia starts during the twenties or early thirties of the life. There will be gradual loss of hair noticed from vertex (center of head facing sky) and temporal regions (sides). This process of falling hair may also begin after attaining puberty. The anterior hairline becomes thin or recedes on each side in such a fashion that the forehead becomes high. In course of time, the top of scalp totally becomes devoid of hair. In some cases, it is not the full-scale hair falling but falling at the vertex and receding of hair on both sides of parietal region. In some cases, there is uniform thinning of hair over the top of scalp with no pattern of spot baldness or otherwise. This thinning leads to complete baldness later.

The rate of falling hair varies from person to person. In the first stage, there will be sudden loss of hair in the twenties and this process of hair falling goes on slowly in coming number of years. The pattern of such hair falling in twenties and thirties of the life is that the hair falling is not affecting the occipital areas and parietal area. A patient of about twenty-five years came to me with complaint of hair loss from front of head and vertex.

His anxiety was that he was getting married. His father had also faced the same problem and he knew that it is by heredity. I advised him to wear the wig because there is no method to eliminate the inherited factors. He did not purchase a wig but was satisfied that there is no treatment. He got married and at the age of thirty-seven, he was completely bald at vertex and forehead.

There is a strong inherited factor in balding. This can be either from paternal or matermal side of the family. This affects both male and female but in most of cases of females, they do not inherit complete baldness. The pity is that the medical science does not know the exact mechanism working behind this theme of baldness. The doctors still advice and consol the patients prescribing medicines and oils etc.

I have not seen eunuchs developing baldness. The science might have attributed many reasons for this but practically; we take it as creation of Almighty.

Female Type Alopecia

The loss of hair in females is very much different. It is primarily a telogen type of hair that fall and similar to male baldness. There is no baldness on the vertex or receding hairline on the forehead as found in males. The hair loss in females is of diffused type. There is thinning of hair on the middle of scalp, the vertex area. There might be some amount of frontal hairline receding but not to the extent, the males get it. The most dreadful situation, as thought by females, is getting bunch of hair on the comb and this cannot be taken as hair loss, if it is not in huge quantity. As a matter of fact, the long hair get entangled after washing and while combing them; some of them get pulled mechanically rather than automatic falling due to some disease. There are some conditioning liquids available in the market, which applied after washing make the hair soft and disentangled.

In females also, the genetic predisposition plays a role for alopecia. The reasons given in the male pattern alopecia as above are also applicable to females. During menopause, the hair gets thin at scalp over the vertex and top of head. The same can be seen in old age. Early baldness in young women has been noticed in those women who use too much of cosmetics, go in for frequent change in hair styling and suffer from endocrine disorders like hypothyroidism.

After washing the hair, when one sees the hair on the floor or basin, this may not be hair loss or thinning of hair. It is because some of the hair roots are shedding their old hair and during the course of time, new one will replace these fallen hair and they will be equally strong.

Alopecia Associated With Disease

As stated earlier, the loss of hair of the scalp may be on account of different causes. In some cases, the situation amounts to not more than a disfigurement but in other cases it may be a manifestation of severe systemic disease. It is, therefore, essential that correct diagnosis of the cause of baldness be made.

The falling of hair can be divided into two main categories, diffuse baldness and patchy baldness (alopecia areata).

The diffuse baldness is one that has fall of hair distributed over the whole scalp. There is gradual loss of hair across whole scalp without any itching or scaling present on the scalp. Diffuse alopecia occurs in females for different reasons.

The *patchy baldness* is the one that has hair fall limited to one area of scalp. This is also called *alopecia areata.* The condition involves loss of hair in patches with normal alp, there would not be any growth of hair in the scarred area. his is called **Cicatricial alopecia.**

In the scar tissues, the follicles are absent because of the injury, wounds, burns or infection. Wounds and injuries like heat burns or mechanical trauma result in scarring and skin diseases. After healing of the injury or burns, scars are seen on the skin and one is shocked to find no hair on them. If the scarring area is more, it is really embarrassing for the patient. Besides injuries and burns, there are certain skin diseases also that leave scars. Impetigo lesions that have persisted on one area for long time and have caused epidermal necrosis leave scarring. Similarly; furuncles, chicken pox, kerion and lupus erythematosus cause scarring after they are healed up. Besides scarring there is localized destruction of hair roots, if the area is subjected to X-ray dermatitis, lupus vulgaris, basal cell carcinoma and scleroderma. There is also a rare cause named as 'folliculitis decalvans' in which minute recurring pustules cause atrophy of the hair roots over large irregular areas of the scalp.

There is no treatment known for growing hair on scarring and burn spots. The only precaution is that while getting the hair cut or hair treatment, the hairdresser should be told not to use hair-straightening chemicals that can burn the scar skin because such chemicals contain alkali. Boils can also cause scar tissues.

Endocrine Alopecia and Alopecia Senilis

Those who suffer from thyroid problems get loss of hairs. In **hypothyroidism,** loss of hair is an associated problem. The hair become dry, coarse, brittle and sparse. In **hyper-thyroidism,** the hair becomes extremely fine and sparse. In both the cases, the hair falling takes place slowly over a period of months or years. There may or not be relation between any of the other endocrine disorders and alopecia or thinning of hair but some isolated instances do occur. Some times, oral contraceptives are responsible in some instances of endocrine alopecia and once the oral contraceptives are stopped, the growth of hair restarts gradually. The treatment is in accordance with general disease.

Some doctors are of the opinion that old age is also associated with loss of hair. It is well known that in old age, the metabolism slows down and nutrients fail to reach the follicles. We can say that this is normal wear and tear of body-mechanism that prevents proper functioning of each system and hair is no exception. There is normal thinning of the hair in most of the people attaining the age of fifty five onwards and nothing can be done for re-growth of hair. This sort of hair fall in old age is called **alopecia senilis.**

Syphilitic Alopecia

Syphilitic alopecia is found in early stages of the disease in association with the early skin eruptions, sore throat and generalized adenitis. It is seldom that this type of baldness is complete baldness. In most of the cases, it is diffused. It occurs on the posterior aspect of the scalp and the hair has **moth-eaten appearance.**

Besides falling of hair from the scalp, there is some falling of hair from eyebrows, eyelashes and other parts of the body. Syphilitic alopecia is temporary and the hair grows spontaneously after the skin disease is controlled by the anti-syphilitic treatment. Its distinct appearance like that of moth-eaten makes it specific to identify.

Seborrheic Alopecia

In diffuse alopecia, seborrheic (disturbance of oil glands in the skin) alopecia is a common form. In most of the cases, this type of hair falling starts from the temples and from the vertex, the crown of the head. It is so slow and gradual that affected persons note it only when the hair falling is obvious at the temples and the hair on the crown appear thin. The process of falling of hair continues steadily until finally the whole of the top of head (vertex) is almost hairless. What remains over the head is a band of hair on the temples and occipital area. In the early stage of this kind of alopecia, the condition is always associated with a marked degree of seborrhea, which is generally a familial (pertaining to family) complaint.

Seborrheic alopecia is observed in its complete form in males. In females, it is in limited diffused form. This sort of baldness starts at the age of about twenty years, which is a severe form. This continues and gradually it captures the whole of scalp by ten years or so.

BALD SPOTS
Patchy Alopecia (Alopecia Areata)

Patchy alopecia, as the name indicates, is loss of hair in patches with normal skin on the scalp. As the hair on one patch starts to grow again, another bald patch may develop elsewhere. There are two main categories of patchy alopecia.

Alopecia areata causes considerable embarrassment to the patients. One or more, small round, smooth, white spots entirely denuded of hair appear on the head and threatens to extend its bald area. Some children and women are very sensitive about their appearance having shining bald spot on some portion of head and the embarrassment is so much that they avoid going to schools and market with naked head. Bald spots generally prefer to be on the head but one can see any area of the body having the patchy absence of hair. The baldness usually appears without local sensation. Occasionally, moderate itching or other manifestations may be present.

The skin is apparently sound and the lesions are irregularly distributed but commonly located on the scalp, especially in the occipito-parietal regions. The bald spots are mostly round in shape and the skin is smooth but somewhat depressed at the denuded space. This depression is not because of any atrophy of the skin but due to absence of hair roots that make up large proportions of the scalp. Without any hair root, the skin looks depressed. This surface is not always free of hair and as a rule, there may be some broken hair at the margin of bald spots or scattered here and there on the surface. These short broken hair look like shape similar to that of 'point of exclamation' (!). This sign is the characteristic of the disease. There may be growth of new patches in the area adjoining the bald spot and this development is gradual during the course of disease.

As a matter of fact, the local patches may enlarge their vicinity to a point and then remain stationary for some period. If untreated, the patches extend further. Occasionally the patches of baldness remain stationary. Most of the times, the patches increase by peripheral extension. *The adjoining patches may merge with the individual patch thus making it a larger patch.* This mode of extension of bald area is characteristic of true alopecia areata. The lesions usually keep their rounded or oval shape but they may form irregular shapes by joining with other patches. It is very rare that at one section of the periphery of existing baldness, multiple zigzag extensions in several directions are formed.

In some cases, a typical form of baldness is observed. The *alopecia spreads in a band-like girdle* around the head just with the hairline. Another pattern is *pea to bean-sized patches* that remain white and they resemble scar tissue.

In some cases, the disease may progress until the *entire*

scalp is involved. It is very rare but a possibility that the entire scalp may suddenly become denuded of hair exists when the alopecia areata begins in early age, childhood or when the patchy baldness persists over a long period and the areas get extended in a short time. There is also a possibility that with the occurrence of bald patches on the scalp or even without any baldness on the scalp, the bald patches may appear on the eyebrows, eyelashes, male beard, the axillae, pubes or even the downy surfaces in either sex.

On the patches, there is loss of sensitiveness to irritants. On the border of the spreading patch, one can see very short hair that can be easily pulled out. In exceptional cases, a few short hair may be seen in the central part of the patch. As and when the lesion turns stationary, the short hair seen on the periphery of bald spots and in the central regions of the bald patches disappear. The longer hair are not so easily pulled out and recovery ensues. This may be seen as the spots become smaller from peripheral hair growth, but *in most favorable cases the hair appears all over the patch at once.* The grown new hair is fine and of light color (or even white) and frequently falls out. This condition ensues for a variable period before its further renewal. Next time, it appears to be nearer to the normal shade. The shedding of hair may be repeated a number of times before the hair loss becomes permanent.

Etiology

There is no clear etiology about this disease and variable statements exist. Both sexes at any age may be affected by alopecia areata. It is more prevalent between the ages of ten and thirty years. According to a study, alopecia areata is less in India and Asia and is much more common in Europe. Against the thinking of most of people, this disease is not infectious and no organisms have been found in association with it. However, doctors opine many conceivable ideas to suggest possible causes of this disease. The reasons vary from endocrine upsets, impacted wisdom teeth, local neuritis, focal sepsis, through error of refraction, traumas, malnutrition, nervous shock and so on but no theory has any base or justification to prove as a clear cause.

More appealing theories conceived about this disease by some experts cite two reasons. According to one theory, it is parasitic and contagious and the other theory is that it is trophoneurotic and non-contagious. In his book, *'Diseases of the skin',* **Dr. Frederick M. Dearborn** (B. Jain, 1992 edition), the author has given his experience about etiology, " From my own experience I should say that the contagious variety is more common although it is less prevalent in the United States than in England, Germany and France. Numerous cases demonstrating contagion have been reported such as several children in the same family, ten patrons of one barber, instances where two or more people intimately associated have contacted the disease and outbreaks occurring in schools. The nature of parasite is not definitely decided; many of the European authorities believing that true alopecia areata are related to ringworm. Others describe fungi or micrococci, which have been occasionally found."

Another Doctor **Dr. Hutchinson** claims that ringworm of the scalp in childhood may result in adult alopecia areata. Similarly **Dr. Crocker** held the view that adult alopecia areata is equivalent to ringworm in childhood. The theory of ringworm as the base of alopecia areata is supported in a sense that the countries where alopecia areata is common, cases of ringworm exist side by side.

Dr. Sabouraud believes that this disease is due to the microbacillus that he found in acne, seborrhea and comedo. He considers this disease as an acute form of seborrhea oleosa.

According to **Dr. Robinson**, pathological findings are due to an inflammation in the corium with round cell infiltration and thickening of the vessel-walls of the affected parts. The resulting interference with the nutrition of the hair results in atrophy of the hair producing structures.

My views

Now that we have learned about the causes, let us know what is practically observed. I have handled many cases of alopecia areata. If the symptomatic theory of homeopathy is observed and totality of symptoms is considered, the improvement starts soon after the induction of remedy. If this starts soon, say by fifteen days or so, I take it as a case of skin disease involving ringworm. In case the alopecia areata is of unknown etiology, the time taken for growth of hair is very long and first symptoms of hair regrowth are observed after one month or so, not before that. If the baldness is due to ringworm, it will react to localize application of mixture of coconut oil and camphor also. The result can be seen within seven days.

One thing is to be remembered that older the patient, the larger will be the area of baldness and longer will be the duration of the disease and treatment. It is essential for the homeopath to differentiate between ringworm and alopecia areata. The fact remains that *originating cause of alopecia areata remains a mystery.*

Diagnosis

It is very simple to make a diagnosis of alopecia areata. One can see the smooth, clean, circumscribed area of hairless skin on the scalp. There will be empty follicle mouths visible on the smooth surface. No other disease of the skin can be confounded with it. The only confusion is with that of ringworm on the scalp. *Ringworm patches always present a dirty scaly surface unless they have been recently washed.* There will be some short hair on the ringworm scalp and they appear twisted and fractured. When they are pulled from the follicles, they break off and do not show any root. Small patches of hair loss accompanied with scaling (dandruff-like) of the scalp and stubby broken hair shafts with the area of baldness is typical of scalp ringworm. To make a consolidated decision, it is better to make a microscopic examination although there is very little doubt on ascertaining the conditions of ringworm and alopecia areata. Microscope will distinguish the fungus if suspected.

The only doubt is to find out about the secondary syphilis. In this case, it is necessary to find out the other manifestations of syphilis, which can be affirmed by serological tests. All other cases of alopecia areata are due to scar formation associated with trauma or pre-existing inflammatory conditions and the presence of scar tissue rules out alopecia areata.

To test whether the disease is active or inactive, one has to pull a hair from the margin where the spot ends (periphery of the patch). In case of active baldness, the pulling of hair will be very smooth.

In diseases like syphilis, lupus erythematosis and favus, the baldness caused may be diagnosed by the history of the course antecedent diseases. Circumscribed baldness from injuries to the nervous structures will have the same surface appearance but the absence of characteristic peripheral hair and the difference in the mode of occurrence and extension should make this type plain.

Treatment

There are many types of treatments suggested in allopathy for alopecia areata. It is said that most of the local applications (ointments or lotions) recommended have a counter-irritant action and general measures depend upon the theoretical view, which prevails regarding the cause of disease. There is no proof that this type of baldness in spots responds to any treatment and the surprise is that the growth of hair commences even with or without any treatment. Counter-irritants do not interfere with regrowth and the patient is relieved or satisfied that he or she is using some applicant. The bald patches and their condition are not infectious and there is no need to restrict children from going to school. Use of wigs has no adverse effect on the scalp to prevent growth of hair.

The method employed in each case depends upon the underlying factors. If the clinical signs of a parasitic disease are present, all the methods of local applicants may be helpful but a penetrating parasiticide is essential. Treatment for the ordinary forms is to clean the affected area and whole of scalp with the help of medicated soaps and shampoos and the scalp be dried quickly. Some doctors advised application of antiparasitic lotion (lactic acid, carbolic acid, formalin or diluted alcohol) and chloroform (chrysarobin as a saturated solution in chloroform) on cleaned area. The most useful applicant in Indian conditions is mixture of coconut oil (10 ml) to one tablet of ordinary camphor (Kapoor). Some of the above applicants are available in ointments.

In homeopathy, the treatment is different and will be discussed in therapeutic and repertory chapters.

Prognosis

There is no need to be dreadful about the disease if the patient is up to the age of forty. The bald patches developed under the age of about forty years are expected to grow in spontaneously after a longer or shorter period up to several years. *It is the multiple patches that take longer time to grow than the single patches of baldness.* If the patches are located near the margin of hair or near the occipital area, there may be delay in regrowth as compared to the single patches.

In case of total alopecia, when the head is totally devoid of hair, the prognosis is doubtful and the same is the doubt about the isolated patches occurring after the age of forty. The growth rate of hair after the age of forty gets slow and hence takes more time.

Initially when the regrowth of hair takes place, the hair observed is thin, downy and at times white but gradually they become thicker and pigmented. If the pigment formation is not starting, it is almost certain that the regrown white hair will fall out again in a short time.

The patchy baldness is a disease that repeats or reoccurs. In several cases, growth of hair may take place side by side with the development of new bald patches on almost adjoining area. It is also common to see that regrowth of hair is taking place on one side of patch and at the same time, there is a continued fall of hair on the opposite margin of the same patch. When the skin has become atrophic after a long time of one year or so, there is little hope of recovery. No time limit can be judged for recovery even in ordinary cases. In cases of nerve disturbance, the hair usually grows again but most of the time, it is abnormal in color. In perfect orbicular type (circular), re-growth of hair should not be expected very soon.

PREMATURE FALLING OF HAIR
Alopecia premature

Premature loss of hair or baldness is hair loss that occur before stipulated age. It occurs without any cause (idiopathic) and it is symptomatic as well.

1. **Idiopathic alopecia premature :** It may occur at any age but rarely before the thirtieth year. One can compare it with senile atrophy that is without any known cause and beyond heredity. Most of the times, it attacks males. In cases of alopecia premature, the loss of hair is noted more than usual- shedding and one notices it on comb or pillows. The hair falling starts from temples and vertex and although the hair may re-grow, it is thin or less vigorous until it ceases to appear. The hairline at the sides of the forehead slowly goes on receding while center of forehead retains the hair for some time. The appearance of the forehead will be like an arch. In some cases, the entire length of hair on temples and forehead recede in a straight line and the forehead shines without hair. In other cases, the hair lose their strong appearance and go on thinning over the whole of crown along with thinning at temples or thin hair extend their regime from vertex forward. Either of the stated preliminary processes occurs and finally baldness on the head is noted under symmetrical condition of the progressive state of this alopecia being untreated, gradual thinning of the hair, left on the scalp, ensues. This process of balding is never rapid and it is very seldom that the hair loss is replaced by growing of gray hair. There is no fast rule for all the growth and falling of hair and it depends upon individual to individual. But most of the times, it is seen that the sides and back of the head remains unaffected.

2. **Symptomatic alopecia premature :** The baldness may be permanent or temporary and all this depends upon

the nature of alopecia along with local and general etiological factors. In this type of alopecia, there has to be a cause. **In case of permanent loss of hair,** there may be local lesions of lupus erythematosis, scleroderma, syphilis, kerion, favus and folliculitis.

In case of temporary hair loss, it may be from localized eczema, psoriasis, some parasitic affections, erysipelas or superficial injuries, typhoid, small pox, excessive drugs intake, abuse of mercury, diabetes, syphilis, leprosy, tensions and worries or mental shocks. The prominent feature of temporary hair loss is that it occurs not during the course of a disease but during the convalescence period. In most of the cases, baldness is temporary and its symptom is thinning of the hair at scalp and other hairy parts. The fall of hair may be rapid, or slow and persistent.

Etiopathology

In idiopathic premature alopecia, the reason of hair fall is heredity in about fifty percent of all cases in males and much larger percentage in females. The amazing feature is that the females are less affected with baldness than men because of abundance of fat in their scalps and lighter and looser covering usually worn by them. Women also take great care of hair in comparison to men. On the other hand, males wash their hair daily and many of them apply soaps also daily. This contributes to alopecia among men. It is also seen that those who do more of brainwork and are intellectuals are more affected by this alopecia.

Metro life full of crowds, pollution, excessive meat- diet, lack of exercise, are all predisposition causes for symptomatic alopecia. Gout and heredity are also important causes of symptomatic alopecia. This type of leading life makes them more prone to some parasitic affection as well. It is also noted that urbane who lead busy life and congested routine work, fall pray to baldness than their counterpart in country life. Pathologically this condition is essentially one of atrophy, both of the connective tissues and the hair growing structures, for want of blood supply to hair- roots.

Treatment

Employing correct nutrition, regular exercise, local care of scalp and washing the hair at proper intervals may arrest the condition of alopecia. Local conditions may be treated specifically. One should avoid frequent washing of hair, if there is no dandruff. Use of hard shampoos to clean the scalp should be avoided. Some young men are in the habit of wetting the hair before combing so as to set the hair at desired level of head and make the hair- style. This should not be done. The combs and brushes should be used individually and these are not to be shared with other persons of the family. Each one should have his or her individual set of combs or brushes. The head covering should only be used when going out in the sun or rains. The caps, hats or cloth covers should be light and well ventilated. Fresh air and light are most important for promoting the vigor of hair. Wearing tight clips, artificial hair, curling the hair and use of hair dryer should be avoided.

Massage of scalp is one of the best methods to correct alopecia. It should be done with light hands for two to three minutes every day and every night. Exercise of the neck along with massage is useful for increasing blood circulation of the scalp. Exercise includes turning head to right side and then to left side for at least five times. Cleaning and washing with any non-irritating shampoo or soap hair every week or twice a week is essential in Indian climatic conditions. After washing, complete drying (natural) is a must and then oil can be applied.

Prognosis

The most unfavorable features leading to early baldness are marked hereditary tendency and atrophy of hair follicles. In many cases of idiopathic variety in its early stage and other cases of symptomatic forms, the disease is curable and the hair falling comes to a standstill position (arrested) by suitable treatment. In case of hereditary background, the prognosis is bad. Nothing much can be done.

Alopecia Congenita

Congenita or congenital means a condition that is existing right from birth or hereditary. Congenital alopecia is a rare occurrence and generally it is temporary. In this condition, the hair loss may be general, in circumscribed areas, with retarded hair growth or with scanty hair growth in character. It is also a condition when there is delayed growth of hair and this delay is associated with defective growth of nails, teeth and other bone structures. When the child suffers from congenital alopecia, the hair grows after a gap of weeks, months or years. In some cases, they do not grow at all and the condition remains permanent. Congenital alopecia is also known as Alopecia Adnata.

Etiology

As already said and as the name of disease suggests, it is apparent that the disease is hereditary. In a family, it is seen that this type of alopecia exists in brothers and sisters but occasionally in their parents. Under such conditions, very little clues can be found from a pathological study except defects in nutrition, incomplete basic development of cutaneous structures and hair follicles.

Treatment

No treatment is feasible but in homeopathy, some medicines may work and they are deep acting, given on constitutional aspects. In most of the cases, the failure is faced as in the case of alopecia premature.

Prognosis

Prognosis is poor and unsatisfactory. In few cases, some sort of hair develops but they look more like artificial hair than real.

Senile Alopecia

Senile (old age weakness) baldness is a part of life, general atrophic changes due to old age. There is no fixed age or exact period of life for senile alopecia to start. Time for alopecia senilis depends upon wear out of tissues and this is highly variable from person to person. As in the case of alopecia premature, almost same conditions and causes are applicable here in senile alopecia. Some doctors are of the opinion that senile alopecia starts its first symptom or sign after the age of forty.

Its onset is from the vertex where the hair go on thinning and then disappear. This trend of thinning and disappearing extends or spreads forward and backward until the whole of crown is affected in a nice symmetry. Then it looks like general thinning of hair that remains constant for few years before total baldness captures. Senile alopecia does not hesitate to approach eyebrows as in alopecia premature. The remains of hairs can be seen on the posterior and lateral region of the head because of greater thickness of the scalp at these areas. Males are more prone to this alopecia and females experience thinning rather than total baldness. In senile alopecia, graying of hair either accompanies or may precede it.

Etio-pathology
Seborrhea is a commonly associated condition in senile alopecia just like alopecia premature. Along with this, any underlying causes, hasten general atrophy thus triggering senile alopecia. The pathological effect of atrophy of the skin and subcutaneous tissues interfere with vascular supply to the hair follicles and reduce the hair growth.

Prognosis and Treatment
Once the atrophic stage starts, the prognosis is bad. The thin and adherent scalp with tissue losses, the defect in vision and hearing, loss of teeth are common old age problems. Once all these processes start, they are irreversible. A retrieval of gone hairs is similarly not possible. No treatment is possible but some precautions as suggested under alopecia premature can arrest hair fall to some extent.

Process of General Thinning or Balding
We have earlier discussed about the dihydrotesosterone in male pattern hair loss. When the dihydrotesosterone has been manufactured, it will be present in the surface sebum (a type of grease). Everyone secretes surface sebum from the sebum

glands present through skin tissues. When a hair has fallen, this dihydrotesosterone will enter the follicle (hole in the scalp from which the hair erupt). Once inside the follicle, there is bound to be chemical reactions which slowly makes the hair weak. There will be new growth of hair but this hair will be finer than the original. When this new fine hair is later shed, the dihydrotesosterone again weakens the follicle and the root further. The next hair grown will be thinner and finer. The process of hair getting thinner and thinner comes to such a stage that there is no growth left due to minute structure at the hair root. If this happens over an area where finer hair has diminished to non-existing stage, the area looks bald.

By inspecting the fine hair growing on the vertex and on the forehead of a man, the doctor can visualize the incoming baldness, if the forehead hair are finer than the hair on the sides of the head. A professional hairdresser can tell this difference and predict the coming baldness.

Excessive Oil And Alopecia

There is a belief or a study that excessive oil in the hair brings more of baldness both in men and women. According to this study, the oil or sebum in the root of hair clogs the pores of scalp and obstructs the follicle growth. A time comes when the hair root is suffocated or asphyxiated due to excessive sebum and this makes it difficult for new hair to grow.

A man has a straight-up growth pattern of hair on his scalp with the result that the oil released from the scalp has no route or place to drain out. This makes the sebum return to the place wherefrom it came. As a result, the sebum does not clean up and it becomes a wax, which clogs the pores. When a hair is shed, its successor cannot come out. It becomes weak and remains under the scalp. Even if the weak hair manages to push through the wax-barrier, it is so fine that it breaks on slight pulling or fall out while massaging. Such type of alopecia is more in men.

On the other hand, a woman has a different set up of hair pattern. Their hair are long and excessive sebum can roll down the hair shaft towards the end. Excessive oily hair on the women-scalp do not affect the scalp to become waxy. The oil-alopecia is less in women.

Some General Causes of Hair Falling (Alopecia)

1. **The heredity :** A great lot depends on the genes, we inherit for hair growth like thick, thin, fine, straight, curly, wavy or sparse.

2. **Age :** The ageing.

3. **Hormones :** The imbalance of hormones as in thyroid disorders, diabetes, pregnancy, contraception by use of birth control pills and menopause.

4. **Infectious disease :** Some infectious diseases and pro-longed illness, (bacterial, viral or fungal infections, internal diseases, high fever, influenza, pneumonia or typhoid).

5. **Mental state :** Mental or nervous disorders, worries, tensions.

6. **Blood supply :** Poor blood flow to the scalp due to excessive worries or other diseases.

7. **Nutrients :** Insufficient nutrients in the blood.

8. **Excretory products :** Poor drainage of waste products through the lymphatic systems.

9. **Medicines and toxic substances :** Chemical therapies, taking of cortisone for acne, or accutane, an anti-acne medication derived from vitamin A, calcium blockers for controlling high blood pressure, cholesterol lowering drugs or drugs for treating scars and medicines for cancer.

10. **Injuries & Accidents :** The injuries and accidents involving the scalp including pulling of hair too much in styling the hair like ponytail or pigtail. The prolonged pulling creates a pressure on the roots and the hair fall at particular spots of pull.

11. **Radiation :** Exposure to chemotherapy, radiation, etc.

12. **Excessive oily hair:** (See the note below)

Note :

Whenever some medicine is prescribed by your doctor for any other problem other than hair, it is better to enquire from the doctor about the side effects of the medicine and its effect on hair.

13. **Menopause :** Menopause is a condition when there is imbalance of hormones and ageing starts. The production of female hormone, estrogen, starts slow working and hence the hair fall.

14. **Pregnancy :** During pregnancy, the hair growth increases due to active and increased endocrine glands-functioning to meet extra demand. After the childbirth, there is irregular thyroid functioning and new life style for the mother. This hair loss is for about two months and the growth becomes normal after that.

Any grouping of two or more causes written above can aggravate the hair loss.

Some Avoidable Causes that Trigger Hair Falling

1. Daily washing or frequent washing of hair with harsh shampoo or hard soaps having chemicals (some dermatologists do not agree that frequent use of

shampoo triggers hair falling. That is why I have used harsh shampoos and hard soaps.).

2. Hard combing of hair, frequent combing of hair.
3. Frequent tightening of hair, frequent pulling of hair.
4. Personal hair styling like use of hot comb, curling iron or blow dryer can make the hair brittle and break.
5. Coloring and dyeing the hair frequently.
6. Wearing a helmet for a longer period everyday.
7. Excessive worries, stress and tensions.
8. Long and frequent journeys by bus, train and passing through variable temperatures and climates (going to foreign lands where climatic temperature difference is more).
9. Lack of vitamins and minerals.
10. Wounds, burns and scarring.
11. Use of scented and branded oils, shampoos and changing them frequently.
12. Not sticking to use of conventional oils on the head (mustard, coconut etc. or the oils being used by individuals from childhood) and changing to variety of scented oils.

When you ask a doctor about the cause of falling of hair, he would offer different causes and each doctor has his own views about it. Doctors take this falling of hair as a general trade enquiry and avoid giving a particular cause. They would cite varied causes of hair falling. On the other hand, if you consult some beauty parlor or professional hair expert, a trichologist, he will give a different opinion about the cause of hair falling. His reasons will have a definite statement about the brand of oil or shampoo that will rescue you from falling of hair. The same is the case with some company's consultant, who manufactures the oils or shampoo or soap and claim care or prevention of falling of hair with their brand. Their main purpose is to sell their product and not to convince you about the cause of falling hair.

A Word of Consolation for Balding Males

Male pattern baldness is the cause of worry for many men. This pattern of falling of hair starts with a receding hairline that gets thin at the top of head in an 'U' shape. During this formation, the hair follicles shrink with each new growth cycle. This male pattern baldness is for those who are genetically predisposed. It is the male hormone androgen that is activated in the body after one achieves puberty. It is again the same hormone androgen that causes destruction of hair follicles after some years due to genetic factor. The male pattern baldness is always progressive and can never be reversed. There are claims by some experts that the progressive baldness cannot be reversed but restricted to one place by use of hormone therapy. Hormone therapy has some side effects too and those should not be forgotten when going in for this.

Keeping a baldhead has become an order of the day. It has been made a ritual of fashion these days, as many famous film personalities, growing old, are intentionally maintaining no growth of hair on their heads to show they are still young with no gray hair. Those who have done it feel very comfortable, as they make statements. There are many young sportsmen, actors and other celebrities who are deliberately shaving their head and adopting baldheads to exhibit that full growth of hair on the head is not the sign of youth or masculinity. It is the baldness that brings charm to the youth and personality. Ironically, it is also said that those having male pattern baldness own more of wealth and are supposed to be rich. This is not found true and remains a proverb only in the countryside.

Permanent Baldness

The heredity is responsible for permanent baldness. This baldness is shoe shaped on the head and sometimes it is called male pattern baldness.

Some hair-experts (Trichologists—a professional who does the study of hair and its diseases) claim that there is a natural treatment available in the market called 'Seranoa Complex'. It is derived from horsetail plant and showed good results of re-growth of hair in about fifty percent of cases.

Means of Treatment

1. **Wearing wig :** There is one simple way to avoid baldness and it is covering the baldhead with a wig. Wearing wig is easy and is quite popular in western countries. There was one popular actor known for his rich dialogue-delivery in films, who used to wear wig right from his youth to the end of his film-career. Wigs are available in the market with different patterns and various styles of hair fixed on them. They can be fitted to any size of head and are available according to small, medium and large size heads. Their cost is according to the quality of hair and cap that holds the hair.

2. **Hair implantation, non-surgical (Artificial Patch) :** Non-surgical hair implantation is an effective method of having hair-filled head. It takes about three hours to fix the artificial hair. The area of scalp requiring hair implantation is measured and a patch is made. Here a sort of pattern or template is put on the scalp having no hair. With the help of some chemicals, a mould is made and a monofilament of similar size of mould is taken. In this filament- holes, the hair matching the texture of the

hair of person are fixed. These hair are made of keratin. It is a very fine art work to fix the hair and this technique is called *silicon winding*. This is now fixed firmly on the scalp of the person requiring implantation with the help of some adhesive. It is also very difficult to judge whether the hair are real or implanted on a filament. When the hair beneath the filament grows, the mould has to be removed, the natural hair beneath the filament are then cut and then mould is again fixed with adhesive. People like this type of hair implantation since this needs implantation every two or three months depending upon the hair growth. Even the natural hair needs a cut periodically and hence this is not an additional job.

3. **Hair weaving technique :** The first procedure of taking a mould is same as done in hair implantation stated above. The difference is that the artificial hair are adhered/weaved to the natural hair. The only problem is that the hair look dense and strangled. This strangulation then leads to breaking when combed harshly. The result is alopecia areata. This technique is not in vogue now and people prefer hair implantation as stated above than hair weaving.

    There is another method in which strand-by-strand hair replacement is done. The hair are replaced by artificial hair, which match the color, texture and density of original hair. This method is called 'Carefree hair solution'.

4. **Hair microwefting :** Hair microwefting is a method by which the hair are implanted in the bald area of scalp after removing from the area where hair-growth is

dense. In two or three sittings, this job is done. This technique is now available in India and it is applied to both men and women.

5. **Single follicle grafting** : Hair grafting by surgical means is a popular solution of evading baldness. Grafting is done in a small area of hair-bearing scalp. Hair bearing area is moved from one area to another area. Hair follicles from a thickly grown hair area are transplanted to bald areas. This method is called 'Single follicle grafting'.

Baldness is, therefore, no problem if you have enough money to spare for hair microwefting or grafting of hair. Consult a good trichologist (a professional who does the study of hair and its diseases) for checking the male pattern baldness and it is he who can suggest better method suitable to your problem. Getting the address of a good trichologist is easy through internet search.

Total hair transplantation tool (Microsurgical transplantation) is also available with literature and DVD education (USA- Internet site has information about it).

Hair Oils and Medicines Claiming Hair Growth (Balding Males)

In USA and western countries, there appears to be a systematic commercial campaign by many companies that claim hair growth for male pattern baldness. Among these medicines and hair oils, there are few products of importance like 'Gero Vital GH3' (Romania), 'Eucapil-Fluridil', (USA- a non-prescription Derma cosmetic product), 'Advecia'(USA-not a DHT inhibitor), 'Hair regain'(US-DHT inhibitor), 'Regain and Propecia'(US-DHT blockers) and 'Procerin'(Portland- for androgenetic alopecia). DHT is a male hormone and some products claim that with the help of DHT, the baldness can be controlled in males. Some of these product manufacturers also claim that 95 percent of baldness of males is due to genetic factors.

Affluent class of India might be trying these medicines because these firms claim that many actors and actresses are using these products and taking advantage. Most of the products are local applicants and there is no harm in trying them because a bald man has nothing to loose at head. Only thing is that one should be ready to pay heavy cost of the medicines. If someone has interest to try these products, internet site, Google-medicine for hair baldness can show many more sites to guide you.

□□□

Graying of Hair (Canities)

Chapter 3

Graying of Hair (Canities)

1. INTRODUCTION
2. GRAY HAIR IN CHILDREN

Graying of Hair (Canities)

INTRODUCTION

In Ayurveda, the ancient therapy of India, there is a reason given for premature graying of hair. It is in Sanskrit 'shaloka' as follows:

> *"Krodh, shok, sharam krita shariroshma shirogat,*
> *Pitam ch keshan pachti palitam ten jayte"*

The meaning of above 'shalok'states that excessive anger, grief and exertions make the body hot and the heat of body goes up towards head. There in the head, the heat pollutes the 'Pitta' (Bhrajak) and it results in graying of hair.

Graying of hair is a sign of old age which is easily accepted by most of people. Being a natural phenomenon, people make no comment over it. When it occurs before the age of, say, thirty-five years, it is considered premature grayness. Those who get early or premature gray hair are the most disturbed people and it is they who resort to coloring or dying. Graying of hair is an atrophic affection of the hair, characterized by circumscribed or general loss or lack of normal pigments.

Graying of hair is actually determined by the hereditary influence (genetically) and it can start at any age. Graying of hair has been seen in the age group of twenty and thirty and this has to be familial. There is also a difference noted in many families where genetic effect of gray hair is not found in all the members of the family. Males mostly resemble the maternal parents in hair pattern and retain the normal color of hair years longer than those bearing the stronger paternal likeness and less frequently vice-versa.

In some cases, it is due to sun-exposures, defects in bones of scalp and short stature (Rothmund and Thomson Syndrome) or Werner's syndrome in which the person has frequent skin changes, of short stature, is prone to cataract and with small bones of hands. As a matter of fact, the melanogenic contents of the skin are less or decreased. Once the melanin is reduced, the hair become gray.

Chronic sinusitis and chronic cold are also stated to be reasons for early graying. People who wash their hair with warm water frequently also get gray hair but this is not the confirmed opinion of doctors. Graying of hair can also be symptomatic of diseases like syphilis, alopecia areata, peripheral neuroses or leucoderma but it often occurs without any definite relation to any other disease.

In some cases, the grayness of hair appears suddenly while in other cases, it is gradual. Either it affects a small part or become more or less general. The change noted is progressive and permanent. Mostly it starts from the head, the temples and then the beard. It is rare that the beard show grayness earlier to graying of head hair. Other regions of the body hair follow later.

Some times there is sudden graying of hair noted and this may be due to severe mental shocks, fright and grief. A similar temporary condition of gray hair arises from disorders of nervous system or organic brain disease.

You must have seen many characters in films and TV serials wherein there are few patches of hair shown as gray. This condition is called 'Ringed hair'. It is a rare peculiar alternate whitening of short sections of the hair growth while the color of the remaining hair is normal. You must have seen on the screen, a giant popular film personality having 'white' French cut beard and 'black' head hair. If it is real, this is either a rare 'ringed' condition (natural) or coloring of head / beard hair or wearing of wig. In some cases, chemicals used in a number of occupations may cause hair color changes.

Etio-Pathology

Premature greying of hair may be congenital or acquired. Congenital graying of hair is very rare and may be seen as a part of the general absence of pigment in the tissues, a condition known as 'albinism'.

According to Ayurveda, the condition of gray hair is called 'Pilitya' that has psychological reasons like excitement, anger, passion and mental strain. Persons having premature gray hair belong to 'Pitta prakriti.'

Heredity may be a cause in premature graying. We have already given specific causes due to diseases and this need not be repeated here. In natural gray hair, age is the chief cause. In premature graying, the causes may be different but triggering factors may be worry, excessive disappointment, trauma, overwork, and general disturbances of nutrition.

The pathological process is in the nature of a trophoneurosis and lack of pigment produced in the hair or even due to presence of air in the cortex of the hair. These are causal factors.

F-8

Prognosis and Treatment

The graying in patches after the age of thirty-five or forty is a condition that can be called progressive and permanent although a few cases may have return of color. The premature graying of hair can be controlled by homeopathic medicines provided the cause is not congenital. In other cases of premature graying of hair, there is no treatment found except dying of the hair although it is improper to do so. Dyeing is never recommended because continuous coloring or dyeing damage the health of hair.

Gray Hair in Children

Parents get worried when they see one or two hair of their child turn gray. Generally it happens at the age between seven and ten years. One or two gray hair in whole of head is not to be bothered about. If there is continuous turning of black hair into gray, the treatment is essential. The cause is related to either malnutrition, some long -standing fevers or boils, imbalance of hormones, diseased scalp and of course some heredity trait.

Child should be under strict vigilance on nature of oil and shampoo being used. If some hard chemical based shampoo is being used, it should be discarded and herbal shampoo should be used. Similarly, scented oils should be restricted and coconut oil should be used.

I have been treating children on this account and found one prescription very useful for gray hair of children. Along with proper homeopathic remedy, following should be given.

Three to four leaves of 'Tulsi' and three pieces of 'Kali Mirch' (grinded powder) should be taken with water on empty stomach everyday for two months.

Homeopathic Treatment

I have seen very good results of homeopathic medicines especially on young girls and boys upto the age of fourteen years. Although a competent homeopath should be consulted for complete course of treatment yet it would not be out of way to suggest a line of treatment to start with.

Children below ten years of age: give four pills of Acidum phos 200 every week for four weeks.

Children above the age of ten years but below fourteen years: give four pills of Lycopodium 200 every week for four weeks.

After a month of this treatment, there may be some changes in the health or in the state of gray hair i.e. either increase or decrease. This is the time to consult a homeopath and take further treatment.

□□□

Dyeing and Coloring of Hair

Dyeing and Coloring of Hair

COLOR OF the hair is determined by heredity Melanin forms the color of hair. If the melanin is more, the color of hair is dark. When you have crossed the age of forty years or so, the graying (graying means no melanin or less of melanin in the pigments) of hair starts at temples, forehead and at places in strands of hairs. When the graying is gradual and according to the suitable age, it is considered natural. People call it a sign of maturity. There is no need to dye the hair at this stage. Once you start dyeing the hair with hair dye or hair colors, it will be a compelled continued ritual. You will be mentally prepared to do it after every 10-15 days. If you do not dye the hair, you yourself would feel awkward and aged. There is no doubt that dyeing infuses a sort of confidence in the person that he or she is not yet old. In real, it is not true. The mirror to the age is not hair but overall health. People do not consider you old just by gray hair. If there is shine on your face and you appear to be full of healthy looks, the gray hair on your head make no difference. You still own a charming personality. The wrinkles, the deep furrows, lines on sides of mouth, darkness or hollowness around eyes and dim complexion altogether expose everything about getting old.

If you do not dye the grey hair, it is convenient for you to accept your face in the mirror. The changes on the hairline are always gradual and people around you, your friends or relatives are already accustomed with your changed looks. Some intimate friends and your husband or wife may make some comments upon graying of hair but that is all. No body is going to remind you every day that your hair are turning gray. It is upto you to accept this God's gift of aging and maturing. It is you who have to decide whether you need a change in color of hair or are happy with matured age and looks. You cannot decieve yourself by colouring your hair.

Once you start coloring, usually, you cannot stop it. When you decide to stop it after a year or so, you would find that more number of hair have grown gray by constant use of dye. The dye is not separately applied on gray hair but its application is on all hair including your natural black hair. There has to be some impact of dye on natural black hair. The dye is going to disrupt the natural flow of melanin beneath black hair or melanin is going to be polluted by constant mixing up with dye. Although it is not proved scientifically that black hair, when applied with black dye, can turn gray but it cannot be denied that excess of everything is bad either it is a diet, food, medicine or a dye. The black hair adjoining the gray hair have been observed to turn gray rapidly after use of hair-dye. This rapid graying of hair can be avoided if dyeing of hair is not started at all. So, think over before you opt for dyeing/coloring your hair.

Do Not Dye or Color Your Hair When —
- **You are pregnant.**

- During the period of menstruation.
- You have heart problems.
- You have skin affections.
- You have asthma.

Important note about use of dye, colors and oil based products

Irrespective of the kind of dye, color or oil based dyeing products, you follow strictly, the instructions given in the literature (provided with the product). Every product has its different set of instructions and hence use them accordingly.

DYEING / COLORING

When you are in the age group of 20-30 years and the hair turn gray, there is a scope that you would opt for coloring of hair if you are from urban area as per the trend. According to the conventional system of medicine, nothing can be done to turn gray hair to black; we have already discussed this in our section of gray hair. But if it is due to after effect of some disease, there is hope to seek treatment. I have seen many people having premature gray hair reversing to black hair after continuous homeopathic treatment for a year or more. The success rate is hardly ten percent. There is one advantage that further rapid graying of hair ends with the use of homeopathic medicines. Along with homeopathic medicines, some diet control, additional measures and restrictions are included in the treatment rituals to achieve better results. Please note that graying of hair cannot be treated if the cause is genetic disorder. *With homeopathic medicines, the premature hair graying having origin other than genetic, can be delayed but not prevented.*

If you have decided to color your hair, you should start with natural colors instead of going in for chemical dyeing. Generally, premature graying of hair is not in bunches and at random places and this can be easily concealed by use of natural dye. Natural dye is 'Henna'. Chemical dyes or chemically treated colors are not good for the health of your hair. Chemical dyes or colors have a toxic base and these can result in allergies and irritation of skin. A skin test of sensitivity is necessary before dyeing the hair. The instructions for conducting skin test are briefed on each pack of good branded dye.

Generally a pack of dye has two bottles in it. One bottle has the dye and the other bottle has peroxide. Peroxide helps the color to go deeply into the bottom of the hair shaft. It is a transporter like alcohol and lengthens the life of color. Once applied, the color does not fade away even if the hair is wash. Further application of color or dye is needed when the roots of the hair show white strands. Peroxide makes the hair dry and porous and professionals who dye the hair in saloon condition the hair after dyeing. To avoid this problem, some manufacturers have produced dyes or colors without peroxide.

If better results of color or dye are needed, one should get the dyeing done from a professional beauty parlor. Now a day, they color the gray hair in such a way that different colors can be seen in streak by streak of hair through diluting the dye, which give a natural look to the hair.

Skin Sensitivity Test (Patch Test)

- Irrespective to the sensitivity to dye, patch test is essential before dyeing.
- Wash a small area of skin behind your ear-area with soap and water and let it dry.
- If you are using powder dye, mix little powder with some

water and apply this mixture on the washed and cleaned area behind the ear. Allow it to dry.

- If you are using liquid dye, mix one drop each of dyeing agents from each of bottle and apply on the cleaned area behind the ear. Allow it to dry.
- Wash this patch of application after 24 hours.
- In case, you do not experience any irritation, itching, swelling, inflammation or redness on or around the area of dye application, you can use the dye.
- In each application of dye or repetition of coloring, this test is essential because every pack of dye may have different brand, batch number and date of manufacturing.
- If you get some of the above symptoms, better consult a dermatologist or a trichologist in beauty parlors.
- In case, you already have some skin eruptions, erosions, abrasions or diseased condition / injuries on the scalp or the adjacent areas before dyeing the hair, better not to use dye and consult the doctor.

If you get a rash on skin after patch test, treat it at home first
- Mix about 100 gms of salt in fresh water.
- Apply this mixture with a soft piece of cloth on the affected part of skin where patch test was undertaken. Do it at least ten times.
- Repeat this application of mixture after every fifteen minutes for about an hour.
- In case of no relief, consult a doctor.

DYEING OF HAIR
Hair-dyes
Dyeing hair at home is an easy procedure and instructions to

do so are written on every pack of dye available in the market. Various colors of dyes are used. The most popular colors are black, natural brown and dark brown. Two types of dyes are available in the market, liquid and dry powder. Some dyes are also shampoo based. On almost every brand of dye, the manufacturers write permanent hair dye. This means that the color, the dye imparts on the hair, is permanent but after the hair grows, the roots of the hair are naturally gray but the stem is still dyed black. It will remain black due to effect of permanent dye until the grayness from beneath the hair overlaps the blackness. When the growth reaches its optimum length, the gray color is visible. This means that on grown gray roots, further application of dye is essential for uniform color maintenance. Some good manufacturers of dye claim that no parting of hair is required while application of the dye and say that dye spreads evenly through the hairs right up to roots.

Liquid dye has two bottles from which equal quantity of liquid is poured out from each bottle and mixed together. One bottle contains the dyeing agent para-phenylenediamine and the other bottle has hydrogen peroxide. The concentration and quantity required for making the mixture is shown in the literature provided with each pack of dye / product. In a good powder dye, the contents of para-phenylenediamine is eight percent and comes to one percent concentration after diluting with stated quantity of water. The powder in definite measure is mixed with lukewarm water, the quantity of which is to be corrected by a plastic measuring can provided with the dye. Some dye manufacturers provide a plastic cup with marked lines (marker) for measuring the quantity needed. Some manufacturers have a single bottle applicant in powder. In some products, the plastic gloves are also provided so that your fingers do not get stained while applying the dye.

Method of Application

- Try a patch test first before application of dye (hypersensitivity test).
- Apply a drop of dye on the back skin of your ear to see weather it produces any allergy or rashes.
- If the dye is suitable, wash you hair to make them oil free.
- Dry hair in the natural way without use of dryer or heater.
- Prepare the dye as per instruction manual and apply the dye on hair, parting the hair in section.
- Let the dye dry for 30 to 45 minutes.
- Wash the hair with shampoo.
- *Never use dye on the eyelashes and eyebrows. It may cause serious damage to eyes , even to the extent of blindness.*

Oil Based Products (Dye)

Dyeing the hair with the help of oils containing dyeing agents is an old method and a product named 'Loma' oil was available in the market in fifties and sixties of the twentieth century. This oil-based product was to be used daily. Now, new oil and herbal-based products with chemicals and colors have come in the market. Oil products of various companies are in use now. It is claimed that no ammonia or peroxide or artificial chemical colors are used in oil-based products.

Many brands of 'Kesh Kala' oils are available in the market. In adopting this method of dyeing, patch test is essential. Patch test is same as detailed before in skin sensitivity test. The oil is not to be used on eyebrows and eye lashes.

Normally, the coloring oils have constituents like P.P.D. liquid paraffin, Cetostearyl alcohol, Sodium lauryl sulphate,

E.D.T.A. disodium, Resorcinol, Propylene glycol, herbal extracts, preservative and perfumes in varying degrees from brand to brand of oils.

Method of Application

- In this method, oil-containing dyeing chemical agents is applied on the hair after washing the hair and drying them.
- The oil is applied and after one hour of oil application, hair are washed with shampoo. In some oil-dye products, it is instructed that oil should remain in the scalp for a day and then before going to bed, the hair should be washed.
- For the next two days, this oil application procedure is to be repeated in the above manner.
- Normally after three applications, the color of hair changes from gray to black or brown as per the color code of the hair oil.
- Once you got the color you desired, the oil application is stopped.
- The oil application will again be required when new streaks of gray hair grow from beneath the scalp. The procedure is same and the oil is to be applied for three or four days till the dyeing effect comes on the hair.
- The oil is to be used preferably wearing gloves on hands so that it does not stain the palms.
- In case, the oil is used with bare hands, it is advised to wash the hands with soap immediately after application.
- If there are some types of eruptions on the fingers or palms, the oil is to be applied on the hair wearing gloves.

- In some brands, the oil can be applied at night after usual washing the hair so that there is no dust in the hair. The oil is left overnight on the scalp and in the morning, the hair are washed with shampoo. A plastic cap or some cotton piece of cloth is worn on the head so that the oil remains in the hair and does not stain the pillow covers.

Henna (Lawsonia inermis-Mehndi)

Leaves of henna (a tropical plant) are best known for their hair and skin dyeing properties. Henna is also known for its therapeutic nature to act as anti-fungal agent. If used in a proper method, it provides a brownish tinge to the hair and covers the gray hair as a coating. *Henna is the oldest vegetable dye that does not change the structure of the hair.* It takes long time to enrich the color of henna on the hair because it is gentle to the hair, unlike chemical dyes. If the chemical dyes have been used in the past and one wishes to change to vegetable dye, it takes still longer time for henna to create a coating of its natural color on the hair. Henna is non-toxic. Gloves would be needed to avoid stains of henna on hand. If you can afford going to beauty parlors for coloring your hair with henna, it would be better because they know the exact technique for different types of hair and condition them before dyeing.

In case, you decide to color the hair with henna at home, here is the procedure.

First Method

- Apply oil by gentle massaging the hair at night, one day before the application of 'Mehndi.'

- Mix three-table spoon full of 'Mehndi' in water to make it a paste (for short hair). By the length of hair needing coloring, one can judge the exact quantity of 'Mehndi' required.
- Mix one teaspoon of coffee and one tablespoon of 'Katha' (Catechus) in it for bringing a dark shade.
- If a bluish tinge is needed in the hair, you can mix indigo.
- Leave this mixture in an iron pan over night.
- It would fetch better results if 'Mehndi' mixture were left in iron pan for at least 16 hours.
- If you want a reddish color on hair, do not add coffee or catechus.
- Wash your hair with some herbal shampoo.
- Dry the hair in natural way (not by dryer or heater).
- Part your hair turn by turn and apply the mixture.
- Allow the mixture to dry up and after completely drying, allow another 30 minutes recess time. Generally three hours of application of 'henna' gives a good result of color. Wash the hair without use of any soap or shampoo.
- Dry the hair in natural way.
- Repeat this procedure after every 10-15 days depending upon the rate of growth of your hair and appearance of gray hair at roots.

Second Method

- Apply oil by gentle massaging the hair at night, one day before the application of 'Mehndi.'
- Mix about 50 gms of 'henna' powder, 25 gms each of 'amla' powder and 'reetha' powder and half teaspoonful of coffee in some milk. Make a paste in the

morning.
- Leave this mixture for about two hours in an iron pan.
- Wash and dry your hair.
- Apply the mixture on the hair and leave it in the hair for three hours so that mixture dries up.
- Wash the hair without use of any soap or shampoo.
- Repeat this application after every three days till you have dyed the hair for four times. Total washing with mixture is four times and then no dyeing of hair for fifteen days. Now apply this mixture once in fifteen days depending upon the growth of gray hair roots.

Third Method
- Mix enough 'henna' in lukewarm water to make a paste.
- Add one teaspoon of limejuice.
- Add indigo half the quantity of henna.
- Add two teaspoons of 'amla' powder.
- Let the mixture stand for one hour so as to dissolve.
- Shampoo the hair and dry them.
- Apply the mixture on hair and let it remain for an hour or so and then shampoo your hair.

Application of 'henna' when the hair have not started getting gray
- When your hair have not started getting gray but you desire to color your hair, here is a preparation that would condition your hair in an excellent way.
- Take two to three tablespoonful of 'henna' powder according to the length of hair.
- Rinse about hundred grams of 'amla' in a cup of water

in the night.
- Leave this mixture for a night and in the morning grind the 'amla'. Do not throw the water in which 'amla' was kept overnight.
- Mix this amla paste with henna powder.
- Add juice of one lemon in it and two to three teaspoonful of coffee powder.
- Now take the left over water of 'amla' and add it in grinded 'henna', 'amla' and coffee mixture so as to make a paste.
- Apply this paste over hair and let it be remained for two hours.
- Wash the hair and you will find shinning, bright and black-brown hair.

'Amla'

Take 'Amla' powder and mix it with water to make a paste. Apply this paste over the hair and let it remain on the hair for half an hour. Wash the hair now. This procedure has to be repeated thrice a week and it acts like a good coloring agent for men and women having short hair. The falling of hair is also controlled by this application.

Tea leaves

Tea leaves have tannin, which is well known for dyeing properties but it has to be in combination with some other related synergistic herb. People mostly use tea leaves with 'henna' powder. In the second method of use of henna as a hair dye as described earlier, there coffee is mentioned. In place of coffee, if tea leaves are used, it gives equally good result. The method of application is same. Instead of coffee, make a decoction of tea leaves. For this, you have to boil two tablespoon of tea leaves in 100 ml. of water. When the water is reduced to 25 ml., this is decoction of tea and it has to be added with the rest of combination of 'henna' and 'amla' as stated in the second method above.

Walnut Shells or Bark

- Use of walnut shells for coloring the hair is an olden method. It colors the hair in a gradual way and not abruptly. Constant dyeing with shells gives good result. The procedure is lengthy and hence people do not opt for it.
- Put some walnut shells in iron vessel (mortar) and water in it to see that the shells are inside the water.
- Add a pinch of salt in this.
- Let it stand for three to four days.
- Now add water four times the quantity of existing mixture and let it boil for at least three hours. Keep on adding water as it evaporates on boiling. Let it cool down.
- Take out the shells from the mixture and press them after enveloping them in a piece of cloth. Twist the cloth to take out dark extract of shells. Put this extract back in the water from which shells were taken out.
- Boil this mixture now for some time to reduce the quantity of total mixture.
- Add some alum in this mixture.
- Boil about three to four teaspoonful of tea in about 100 ml of water to make a dark liquid. Add this to the mixture of shell nut.
- Strain the mixture through a cloth for application to the hair.

- Shampoo the hair and let it dry.
- Apply the mixture on the hair wearing a pair of gloves. The mixture is not a paste and hence rinse the hair with the mixture.
- In the first application you will get a yellowish color but after more of application at three to four days interval, you will get the hair a black natural color.

Hirakasees (Ferrous Sulphate)

Hirakasees is ferrous suphate salt that has properties of natural dyeing when used in combination with the herbs of similar properties. I have observed professional experts doing dyeing jobs use 'hirakasees' with 'henna', tealeaves and coffee. 'Hirakasees' is generally known for its use as a paste (mixed with water) in the night and rinsing the hair in the morning. It ensures a type of mask on the gray hair but has to be repeated every week.

Kali Mehndi

You must have read or heard about 'Kali Mehndi' or 'Black Henna' available in the market. There is no pure or natural 'Mehndi' that can give black tinge. 'Mehndi' has its natural tinge of red and not black. The brand name of black 'mehndi' is not pure 'mehndi'. A chemical called Para-phenylenediamine (PP) is mixed in little ratio in natural mehndi and its gives a black tinge. When you purchase any branded 'Kali Mehndi' product, see the printed manual in the packet and you can find the ingredients having the above chemical. If you find any brand without any chemical but with other vegetable (natural) dye, it has to be very safe for hair. Such a product is still to come in the market.

Having some contents of Para-phenylenediamine in a vegetable dye like 'mehndi' is safer to use than using other dyes having only chemical dyes. Those hair dyes with chemicals are also supposed to be somewhat safe if their contents of PP are less than one percent after dilution and less than eight percent in net contents. In powder dyes like 'Kali Mehndi'available in the market, the Para-phenylenediamine is eight percent and on diluting with water, the concentration comes down to one percent. At a time, full contents are not used for short hair and hence 'Kali Mehndi' is slightly safer than powder dyes having only chemicals. Before use of 'Kali Mehndi', the skin sensitivity test is needed as usual.

HAIR COLORS

It is to be understood that hair colors are not hair paints or dyes. There is a difference between color and dye. The dyeing agent is to make gray color black or brown whereas the coloring of hair is the fashion of the day when some one desires to give a different tinge (orange, golden, yellowish red and so on) to his or her black, brown or gray hair. In both dyes and colors, the key or chief ingredient is again Para-phenylenediamine.

Colors are available in creams and liquids i.e. colorant and developer. Color creams are non-dripping and some people prefer the same. There is a range of shades in colors. They are natural black, soft black, natural brown, light brown, black brown, copper brown, dark mahogany, burgundy etc. Most of the colors claim to contain hair conditioners also.

When you see any color on any object, not to speak of hair only, it is reflection of light on the object that transmits the color. Color has different combinations of reflections of light. If you watch the colors of hair in different light mediums, say in bulb light, sunlight or fluorescent lights, the colors would look different. Hair colors are allotted a definite number by manufacturer, a sort of standardization that counts from one to ten in colors. For example, black color hair will reflect very little light and a blonde would reflect more of light. This reflection of light has been allotted numbers. Color number one is called black and number ten is blonde. This type of standardization applies to all colors and almost all brands mostly available in the market have this numbering.

Under the heading 'Dyeing the Hair' earlier, you have read about 'permanent' dye. Let us be clear about it again that permanent means permanent color so far its color is concerned on the hair shaft. The roots of the hair that are gray or of natural pre-coloring stage remain in the same order without any coloring effect. On the hair shaft where the color has been applied, it does not wash out. This color may fade after some time with sunlight and other climatic effects but cannot be removed. Actually the hair are chemically changed by colors.

Coloring the hair is expensive. One can color the hair without the help of professionals but it is better to *get the colors done from beauty saloons,* which are equipped well with tools and means to color hair. Many color- brands are available in the market that claims good coloring results.

The color that deposits on the hair is called color deposits. This is easy to use and is available for home users. It conditions the hair and colors the hair in one step. With the color, hydrogen peroxide is also supplied (about 3 percent concentration).

Permanent and semi-permanent hair colors. We have already detailed about permanent colors. Semi-permanent color has capability to give color to gray hair and then turn them darker. It does not get lighter whereas permanent colors do get faded. Semi permanent color lasts for some time depending upon the product, permanent colors last longer.

Single process color is the color used by home users themselves and not by professionals. They are easy to use and just unpacked, lifted and deposited on hair in one step. There is not much of difference between color deposits and single process color.

It must be remembered that irrespective of use of colors or dyes, it is essential to re-do the roots of hair every 3 to 4 weeks for ladies having long hair and every 2-3 weeks for gents and ladies having short hair.

Coloring Procedure

- A patch test is essential as is in the case of dyeing of hair.
- Shampoo and towel-dry your hair before using colors.
- The container in which the colorant is poured and the brush or comb should not be of metal. It should be either plastic or glass container.
- Wear pair of gloves on the hands.
- Avoid contact of the color with eyes.
- Do not use the color on eyebrows and eyelashes.
- In case some color goes inside the eye, rinse the eyes immediately.
- If some extra color has stained the adjoining area of margin of hair, wipe it off with cotton after wetting the cotton with water and shampoo.
- The excess contents of color taken out of bottle should not be saved or kept for next application. It should be thrown.
- Keep the color pack out of reach of children.
- While coloring the hair, protect your clothes with some old towel.
- If your hair had been colored with a dye or 'Mehndi',

give at least 15 days gap between dyeing and coloring to get better color.

- If you had permed your hair or straightened your hair, keep a gap of at least three weeks between perm and coloring.
- With every color pack, there is an instruction manual, which should be followed strictly to get the best result.

Care of Hair After Coloring

- After you have got your hair colored, follow the advice of beauty parlors. The professionals advise use of color enhancing shampoos to maintain the color of hair till the roots become gray or color-less and need fresh coloring. **The color-shampoo** helps to keep the color looking good until next application of color. If your intention is not to use color shampoo, use some mild and gentle shampoo to wash your hairs.
- It is better that no oil should be applied on the colored hair for three days so that the oxidation of hair takes place properly.
- The colored hair are not to be exposed much to the sunlight.
- Washing the hair with very hot water is to avoided.
- The water that has much of chlorine is to be avoided for hair washing. In swimming pools, chlorine is added abundantly and this will fade the colors or give a green tinge to your hair, if you take bath frequently in swimming pools. Do not swim bare headed.
- The colors normally make the hair dry. **Hair conditioning** should be done from time to time. Hair conditioners are available in the market.

- Curds mixed with lemon juice gives a good conditioning to hair and its continuous use makes the gray hair black.
- Cleaning and conditioning of hair is well done when the hairs are washed with curds mixed with grinded ten pieces of black pepper, 'kali mirch'. Leave the mixture for 20 minutes on the hair then wash the hair without use of soap or shampoo.

Hair Pack after Coloring or Dyeing

Those ladies who color or dye their hair regularly can use a hair pack so that the health of their hair is maintained. Take about 6 teaspoonful of 'Multani Mitti' in a big jug. Squeeze juice of one lemon and extract of one egg in it. Mix them and then add two teaspoonfuls each of 'Shikakai', 'Amla' and 'Reetha'. Again mix them and add half a cup of beer in it. Now apply this mixture on your hair and wait for an hour. Now shampoo your hair. This conditioning of hair is not to be done on the day of coloring but in between days of next coloring.

Gray Hair Highlighting

In case your hair have started turning gray and they are very few of them, highlighting these gray hair is another method to conceal gray hair in their own way. Such highlighting can be got done from beauty parlors. In this procedure, only gray hair are touched in a lighter color than the natural color of your hair. In another method, gray hair are colored lighter than the color of other hair that are colored darker than the color of gray hair. Such an appearance of hair is called glamorous. You can find many TV actresses with their hair colored in two different shades.

Follow-up Coloring

As a matter of fact there is no thumb ruel for this. It depends upon the rate of growth of hair and it varies from person to person. Ladies have long hair and the white-growth at the root of hair is not easily visible and it is seen on the margin of head around temples. On an average, monthly dyeing or coloring is supposed to be safe to cover the white growth at hair roots and renew the color on hair shafts.

Selection of Colour

Now this is a tricky question because everyone has his or her own choice. There are different colors to choose. Golden, dark black, dark brown, light brown, yellowish brown, light black and many more mixed colors are available for coloring the hairs. In India, the common colors seen in metro cities are black, light black, brown, golden and dark brown. Multi color is also the fashion of the day. The other day, I saw a girl with brown puffy hair having two or three fine streaks of dark black hair in the middle of head. Selection of color is a choice varying from person to person. One should remember that age factors must be considered before opting for different colors. There has to be an added grace to the personality. If you are young, you can choose dark colors and if you are middle aged, it is wise to wear light colors.

Washing Hair Before Coloring or Dyeing

If you read the instructions of the manufacturers of the colors and dyes, you will find an instruction that the hair should be washed with shampoo so that they are dirt free and the dye or color can originate on the hair soundly. Oil contents, if existing on the hair, may not allow the color to deposit on the hair firmly. If you go to ordinary barber saloons where hair cutting is done, they also do the same. They wash the hair first, dry them and then apply the dye or color. Since I had planned to write a book on hair, I consulted expert professionals running beauty parlors so as to collect the data about hair and associated all job written in the book including the care of hair and accessories needed. You will note that every good professional has developed his own innovative method to conduct the jobs connected with hair. They also maintain a professional secrecy and do not reveal everything in details especially on coloring of hair.

On my enquiry about the washing of hair before coloring, some of them differ and state that no washing is needed. Some customers insist for washing the hair as they had read in the manuals provided with products but most of them leave the whole of procedure to the professionals. The justification for not washing the hair has some rationality. The longevity of the color or dye will be less and they would fade soon because of oil present on the hair. This would mean earlier re-dyeing the hair than the schedule. This would benefit the beauty parlor.

The other justification is that the oil present on the hair, if not washed before dyeing, would protect the skin from bad effects of chemicals in the dye. The effect of dye would be penetrating and severe when the hair are free of oil and dirt. The option about washing the hair or not getting washed before dyeing / coloring is yours.

EFFECTS OF HAIR DYE AND ALLERGY

Hair dyes and hair colors are injurious to the health of scalp and brain. Continuous use of hair dyes for decades has even led to insanity in some cases. Use of hair dye once or twice a month is not stated to be very harmful. Leaving aside this topic of continuous long use of hair dye, in case the allergy occurs on the margin of hair or there is itching after the use of dye or color, homeopathic treatment gives early relief. Those who get such allergies or eczema should take one dose of Sulphur 200 in pills. If this does not give relief, they should consult the homeopath.

Preventive for Dye-Allergy

Those who use dye and color continuously, say every fortnight or month should take one dose of Tuberculinum 200 after every three months.

Herbs and Foods for Health of Hair

Chapter 5

Herbs and Foods for Health of Hair

INTRODUCTION

If you have seen ladies from the countryside living near sea, you must have praised the shine and health of their long hair. The reason is their fish eating habit. Bengalis have a special liking for fish and I have seen most of Bengali men and women having very healthy long hair and seldom you will find them suffering from premature gray hair problem or falling of hair. Similarly, ladies living near coastal areas of Kerala, Orissa, Andhra Pradesh, Goa, Maharashtra, West Bengal and other states have long black hair.

Fish is their prime diet for healthy hair. There is also a part played by heredity. Naturally, from times immemorial, their ancestors have been living in coastal areas and taking fish. Some families consider that taking fish is a vegetarian ritual. The fish is rich in omega-3 fatty acids, which help replenish lost moisture in dry hair.

Women take extra care of their hair than men for obvious reason of glamour and good looks. On the other hand, men

are more exposed to sun heat or other climatic traumas that
spoil the hair grooming. They are not very much careful
about their hair as compared to women, especially in rural
areas. They have to be out to earn a livelihood whereas it is
not essential that every woman is a working woman. Even
women working in open fields of villages never keep their
head open to sun and winds. This offers them protection from
harsh climate. Taking fish twice a week helps in checking
falling of hair, replenish lost hair moisture in dry hair and
produce long hair besides preventing hair to turn gray before
maturity.

With the changing times, there has been a lot of change in
the life style of people. The urbans have switched over to fast
food, concerned more with material luxuries and are always
busy in a self-created race to excel in service or business. In
such a busy life, they have no time to cook their meals
everyday and thus find tin stuff or ready-made food easy to
consume. They have no time for regular exercise and to
exhibit their body fitness, they use cosmetics and dye hair.
Over and above all this, television has made a traumatic effect
on the mind of people and they follow whatever is shown on
it as good for health. There are many other things that could
be discussed for care of health in general but here our topic is
hair. Hair can be saved from the disastrous applicants
available in the market. Today you will find it very common
to see urban young men and women suffering from premature
gray hair and falling of hair. Diseases of premature gray-hair
and falling of hair are uncommon in village- youths because
TV and modern cosmetics have not yet polluted the hearts
there and people are still living in the lap of innocent nature.
If you, a city dweller young man or woman, have confidence,
you can also take the shelter of natural treatment for care of
your hair.

FACTORS AFFECTING HEALTH OF HAIR
1. Food

Food has intimate relation with mind and body. Mind is madeup of the subtle part of the food. In Ayurveda, food is of three kinds; 'Satvik', 'Tamsik' and 'Rajasvic'. 'Satvik' is the diet containing cereals, butter, milk, wheat, cheese, curds, tomatoes, fruits and vegetables. 'Satvik' food gives the mind peace, calm and purity. 'Rajasvic' foods are mixed foods with luxuries of heavy 'masala' and oil and servings with variety of foods. 'Tamsik' foods are meat, onions, garlic, wine, and tobacco. These induce darkness and anger in the minds. Actually different foods affect different areas of mind. It is the head that holds the mind and it is the hair that covers the head. The diet, therefore, plays a vital role in maintaining the health of hair. It is the perfect nutrition that holds key to the health of the hair.

2. Sleep and Rest

Sleep is very necessary for the health of hair. It is the sleep that gives rest to the body. The hair also need rest and immobility. All through the day, the hair are subjected to rough frequent combing, harsh winds, rains, storms, sun- heat, cold and heavy atmospheric pollution. Hairs do not get any rest. In the process of rest and sleep, new cells are formed in place of destroyed cells. It is the resting and sleeping time, which is utilized by the body for growing hair in place of fallen hair. A person gets renewed vigor and energy when he or she wakes up from sleep in the morning. Same is the case with every part of the body including hair. To a great extent the health of hair depends upon sleep and rest. Those who sleep late, watching TV or work in night shifts have been observed to have more diseases of hair.

F- 10

3. Water

About seventy five percent of our body consists of water. Water is very essential for digestion, circulation of blood, overheating of body and health of hair. To keep body fit, at least ten to twelve glasses of water should be taken everyday. Similarly cold water bathing is necessary for the health of hair. A cold bath stimulates the circulation of blood and aids in the elimination of impurities in blood. A good circulation of blood in the head strengthens the hair. Water is a valuable health promoter.

Important note :

Given below are some methods for stopping ailments of hair and it is up to you to check the adaptability and suitability of the method as per your body. If you find some sort of allergy or rashes during constant use of the methods given, you should consult a doctor.

GUIDELINES FOR HEALTHY HAIR

- Stop using soaps and shampoos for cleaning your hair.
- Comb your hair daily at night before going to sleep. The combing is to be done for at least 80-90 times to and fro from root to the end of hair.
- Apply mustard oil or coconut oil on the fingers and massage the scalp thoroughly. In winter, mustard oil is good and in summer, coconut oil should be preferred.
- In the morning, make a mixture of 'Besan' (powdered gram) and water in a vessel then add some curd. Wash your hair with this mixture.
- Those living in villages and small towns can get some fresh earth dug from the fields. Wet it for some time and

wash the hair with this earth. Earth should be from a
good clean field.
- Scented oils and inferior quality oils should not be used.
- Do not change the hair oil frequently.
- Do not apply oil on the scalp till the hair are completely
dry, up to roots.
- Include 'Amla' (Myrobalan- Emblicas officinalis) in your
diet in any form like pickles, raw, vegetable, 'murabba'
etc.
- Take green vegetables, milk and milk products, foods
containing vitamin B, C, D, iron, calcium, iodine and
protein.
- No late night sleeping and early morning walk is
essential for health of hair.

Boils on Scalp
'Kala Jeera'
If there are small crop of boils on the scalp or intense itching or
eruptions with red surroundings, try application of mixture of
powdered 'kala Jeera' and water. Apply this at least twice a day
and you will find the boils gone within seven days.

Graying and Falling of Hair
'Triffla'
- Triffla is a mixture of 'Amla-Behrha-Hararh' available in
the market from any Ayurved chemist shop.
- Take a teaspoon of 'Triffla' powder every night with
lukewarm water or milk.
- Mix two teaspoon of same 'Triffla' and dissolve it in a
glass of water in the night.
- In the morning, filter the mixture with a fine cloth.

- Rinse your hair with this mixture.
- Taking 'Triffla' at night and washing hair with it as stated above should be continued for at least six months.
- Another method is to prepare a grinded mixture of 'Amla', 'Bhringraj', 'Mishri' and 'Kala Til'.
- Take teaspoon of this mixture morning and evening everyday for six months.
- In place of 'Mishri', in the above mixture, 'Gokhru' can also be used.

Falling of Hair and Dandruff
Ist Method
- Take one teaspoon of coconut oil and half teaspoon of lime juice.
- Mix them and apply on the hair with the help of fingers by massaging.
- Leave it for at least one hour and then wash the hair.

IInd Method
- Mix one teaspoon of honey and one teaspoon of onion-juice.
- Apply in the same above manner and wash after an hour.

Dandruff
Procedure
- Make a solution of sugar and water and add lemon in it.
- Apply it on the hair with fingers and do massaging.
- Leave it on the hair for half an hour.
- Wash the hair.

Falling of Hair
Procedure

- Mix two teaspoon of vinegar ('sirka') in one liter of water.
- Wash your hair and dry them.
- Take a teaspoon of vinegar and mix it in a teaspoon of water.
- Apply this mixture on the roots of hair.

Coconut Oil
Regular application of coconut oil on the hair stops falling of hair. It lengthens the hair also.

'Chukandar' (Beet)

- Application of grinded leaf of beet and 'Mehndi' together help remove falling of hair and enhances the growth of hairs.

'Kakrhi' (Cucumber)
Taking cucumber daily helps reduce falling of hair. Its juice can be used for washing the hair to make hair strong. Cucumber has more of sulphur and silica and hence they give life to hair and nails. Take it with its skin and without salt.

'Dahi' (Curd)

- To avoid falling of hair, wash the hair with curds. Apply curds (sour curds is better) on the hair and leave it for 30 minutes.

- Wash it without use of any soap or shampoo.
- Cleaning and conditioning of hair is well done when the hair are washed with curds mixed with grinded ten pieces of black pepper, 'kali mirch'. Leave the mixture for 20 minutes on the hair then wash the hair without using soap or shampoo.

'Patta Gobhi' (Cabbage)

Wash and soak about 50 to 60 gms of leaf of cabbage in warm salty water for some time and eat them raw before meals for some days. It is said that cabbage even removes the habit of falling hair and new hair growth is established.

'Cholai' (Amaranthus Viridis)

Leaves of cholai (cholai saag) are very commonly used in Northern India. Taking 'cholai saag' at least twice in a week prevents falling of hair.

'Amla' (Emblica Officinalis)

Put some dried 'amla' in water and keep it overnight. In the morning rinse your hair with this water after filtering 'amla' out of water with a piece of clean cotton. Rinse your hair with this twice in a week. The roots of your hair will get strengthened and falling of hair will stop.

Alopecia Areata (Falling of Hair in Patches)
Lemon

In the case of alopecia areata (loss of hair in patches), rubbing of lemon every day for a prolonged period helps in growth of hair. Curds mixed with lemon juice gives a good conditioning to hair and its continuous use makes the gray hair black.

'Arhar Daal' (Cajanus Cajan)

Grind 'arhar daal', make a paste with water and apply on the patch of hair loss (alopecia areata) after cleaning the bald spot with water. Leave it for at least half an hour and then sit in the sun next after applying mustard oil on the bald spot for ten to fifteen minutes. Do the same routine for some days.

Dandruff
Amla (Myrobalan / Emblica Officinalis)

In the case of falling hair and dandruff, dried 'amla' may be soaked in water overnight and in the morning, the filtered water of 'amla' be applied on the hair everyday. It will stop dandruff.

'Til' (Sesamum Indicum)

Massaging 'til' oil is good for removing dandruff. After half an hour of this massaging, wrap the hair in hot water soaked towel and leave it there to cool. Repeat this procedure once again and then wash the hair with cold water.

'Dahi' (Curd) and Lemon

- Cut the lemon in two and rub the same on the scalp while squeezing the lemon at times, in between. Leave the application for half an hour and then wash the hair. Let the hair dry.
- Next day, apply curd on the scalp and let it be there for

an hour. Wash the hair after one hour.

- This procedure should be repeated once a week, say Saturday and Sunday. This is one of the best methods to remove dandruff from hair and conditioning the hair.

Coconut Oil, Lemon and 'Reetha'

- Apply coconut oil mixed with some lemon juice on the hair at night. Let it remain there on the hair overnight.
- In the morning, wash your hair with 'reetha' water. For making 'reetha' water, immerse pieces of 'reetha' in lukewarm water for half an hour. Filter the water with cotton cloth and use this water for washing.
- Use this method twice a week and after one month, the dandruff will be over.
- 'Reetha' alone when kept in water overnight serves the purpose by washing the hair with this 'reetha' water in the morning even if you have not oiled your hair at night.

Coconut and 'Kapoor'

Take 100 gm of coconut oil, 4 gms of 'Kapoor'. Mix them and store in a bottle. Massage this oil twice in a day. Wash the hair with lukewarm water after applying half-cut lemon on the scalp. Repeat this thrice in a week to remove dandruff.

Premature Gray Hair
'Tulsi', Basil (Occimum Sanctum)

It is wonderful herb for the health of hair and premature gray hair. The leaves of 'tulsi' and 'amla' powder mixed with some water and its paste should be applied on the hair. After fifteen minutes, wash the hair. Be careful that its contents should not enter the eyes when applying this paste and while washing the hair.

'Til' (Sesamum Indicum)

Eating about half teaspoonful of 'til' (black) every day turns the premature gray hair black 'til' should be preferably taken in winter for three-four months for better results.

'Kali mirch' Black Pepper

- Five pieces of pepper and ten pieces of seeds of 'Sita-Phal' (a fruit) be grinded together with some water to make a paste.
- Mix some 'ghee' in it and apply on the scalp. Wrap the hair with cloth and leave this mixture for the night.
- In the morning, wash the hair. All the head-lice and dandruff will be removed.
- After seven days, this can be repeated. Caution is that while washing the eyes should be closed so that the contents do no enter the eyes.
- Black pepper is also useful to turn premature gray hairs black. Those who consider that their hair have turned gray due to frequent cold and coryza or sinus problem, black pepper is good. Such people should chew 6-8 pieces of pepper in the morning empty stomach and in the evening also. The result can only be seen after continuous use of pepper for a year.

My Views and Experience on Black Pepper

I always advise my patients to use black pepper as a routine while they take homeopathic medicines for premature gray hair. My prescription is that 5 pieces of black pepper should be grinded and taken with water and along with it, 5 'tulsi' leaves should be swallowed with the help of water. I am not sure, which works, the homeopathic medicines or the pepper and tulsi but the results are seen after about six months, if the reason for premature gray hair is frequent cold, coryza and sinusitis.

The Natural Way to Make the Hair Black
Ist method
Take about 100 gms each of 'Amla, Shikakai, Reetha, Bhrigraj, Brahmi, Methi dana, Til' oil and 50 gms of 'Kapoor Kachri'. Grind all of these items (except oil, naturally) into powder separately and then mix them. Now filter it in small sized net so that the powder has no rough contents and it is very thin. Now put this powder in an iron pan and mix 'Til' oil. Add one litre of water in it and boil it over fire till the whole contents become half the total quantity. If the mixture is too thick, you can mix more water and boil. When the mixture is cooled, filter it with net so that the thick residues are removed. Wash your hair without using soap or shampoo. After washing the hair, dry your hair in natural way and apply this mixture on the hair gently with the help of fingers so that it spreads on the whole of scalp. It is better not to apply 'Mehndi' on your hair during the period when you continue application of mixture on hair. Apply this oil daily on the hair except on the day when you wash your hair with shampoo or soap. You will find the hair turning black after few months.

IInd method
One cup of 'Henna' powder, one teaspoonful each of curd,

coffee powder, lemon juice, powdered 'katha', powder of 'Brahmi Buti', 'Amla' powder and 'Pudina' powder should be mixed with water to make a paste. Keep this mixture in iron vessel for two hours. Apply this paste on your hair and let them dry for two hours. Then wash the hair. Apply this mixture twice or at least once a week. Continue this for six months and you will find your hair black.

IIIrd method

Do not wash your hair with shampoo or soap. Grind 'Amla' and mix it with 'Mehndi' powder. Mix this with water and keep it overnight in an iron vessel. In the morning apply this paste on the hair. Repeat this twice a week. After six months, you will see that your premature gray hair have turned black and there is no need for further use of this mixture. Of course the balanced food and nutrition in meals is essential.

IVth method

'Henna' powder and 'Amla' powder should be mixed in some milk to make a paste. Apply this paste over the hair and let it remain on the hair for one hour after which the hair should be washed with lukewarm water. Conduct this practice twice in a week for at least six months.

Removing Head Lice
Neem (Azadirachta Indica)

The leaves of 'neem' tree should be boiled with water and then cooled. Now wash the hair with this water. If the hair have started falling recently, they will stop falling. Repeat this washing every third day for a total of four washings. This washing will also remove head-lice. The caution while washing the hair is that the neem-water should not enter your eyes. Keep your eyes closed while washing.

Juice of Onion

Apply the juice of onion on the head and let it remain for thirty minutes. Wash the hair. Conduct this practice thrice in a week.

'Suhaga and Fitkari' (Boric and Alum)

Grind fifty grams each of 'Suhaga' and 'Fitkari' and mix them. Take two spoonful of this mixture and mix it in a mug of water. Wash your hair with this water every third or fourth day.

Kerosene oil and Neem

In villages, I have seen ladies applying kerosene oil on the head. The kerosene oil is left overnight on the scalp that is covered with cloth. In the morning, the hair are washed with 'neem' soap. Almost all the lice get killed.

Hair Cuts and After Effects

Hair cut is a common monthly routine for men. Women working and living in cities are not exempted from it. Those who get accustomed to regular hair-cuts and shavings do not have after effects but children are more prone to it. The after effects vary from skin allergies, congestion, redness of face or fear / anxiety, etc. Homeopathy has good medicines to combat such problems. It should be assured that the hair-cuts should be from a barbershop that maintains cleanliness in its equipment and shaves or cuts the hair with a new blade.

Medicines Recommended

— Children, those who are afraid of hair-cuts and refuse to go to barber shop : *Cina maritima 30*, 4 pills three times a day for two days.

— Fear, redness of face, anxiety, heat of head : Give *Glonoinum 30*, 4 pills three times a day for three days.

— Red eruptions over the neck area or surrounding area of hair cutting : *Belladonna 30* in the above manner.

— Diarrhea after hair cutting : *Belladonna 30* in the above manner.

— Earache after hair cutting : *Ledum palustre 30* in the above manner.

— Hardness of hearing or feeling obstruction in ear after haircut : *Ledum palustre 30* in the above manner.

— Stiffness of neck after the haircut : *Belladonna 30* in the above manner.

— Cannot comb smoothly after haircut : *Borax veneta 30* in the above manner.

— Sneezing after haircut : *Silicea terra 30* in the above manner.

— Hair entangle too much after hair cut : *Borax veneta 30* in the above manner.

□□□

Medicines Recommended

Children: those who are afraid of hair-cuts and refuse to go to barber shop : Calm bromatio 30. 4 pills three times a day for two days.

Fear, redness of face, anxiety, heat of head : Give Glonoinum 30, 4 pills three times a day for three days.

Red eruptions over the neck area of surrounding area of hair cutting : Belladonna 30 in the above manner.

Diarrhea after hair cutting : Belladonna 30 in the above manner.

Earache after hair cutting : Ledum palustre 30 in the above manner.

Hardness of hearing or feeling obstruction in ear after haircut : Ledum palustre 30 in the above manner.

Stiffness of neck after the haircut : Belladonna 30 in the above manner.

Cannot comb smoothly after haircut : Salix venata 30 in the above manner.

Sneezing after haircut : Silicea terra 30 in the above manner.

Hair entangle too much after hair cut : Borax ener. 30 in the above manner.

□□□

Care of Hair

Care of Hair

Care of Hair

MEN HAVE never taken care of hair seriously in the past. They were not so conscious about upkeep of their hair. With the changing times from last one decade and with the advent of fashion inducted through media, cinema and television, the men have changed. Businessmen have commercialized the beauty-business and exclusive beauty parlors for men have started functioning in big towns and cities. The hair cut cost that used to be from rupees five to ten has been raised to rupees twenty to one hundred or even more. Hair upkeep is not a concern of females but has been pondered over by males. It has been a concept from the times immemorial that ladies are more conscious about their hair. The elders in the family who teach them about the care of hair and how it adds charms to their beauty and personality. Lengthy and shining mane of hair is indeed appreciated.

Exclude those fashion-crazy and hair-conscious men in urban areas and you will find that men in general, more than eighty percent of whole men-population of India, do not bother about their hair until the hair are captivated by some disease like dandruff, falling of hair and baldness. By the time men realize that the hair need some care, the time to take care is gone. In care of hair, one must remember that amount; color and shine of hair you have got on your crown are the product and result of genetics, your family. Even if you do not care much about your hair, there will not be any serious problem. Cleansing or oiling of hair once or twice a week (if not daily), combing them regularly and toning the scalp with massage are normal care methods and these are sufficient when you are gifted with good normal hair through heredity. Cleansing of hair daily eliminates the debris of dead hair cells (hollows) and helps in the hair growth in proper way. Please note that a basic care of hair is what you need and not a strict discipline or ritual.

Taking care of hairs should be at par with taking care of skin. If you give a massage to your skin, tone it with creams, soaps and conditioners, it remains very good. The same discipline has to be maintained in the case of hair.

USEFUL HINTS FOR CARE OF HAIR
Long Hair
Long hair is an all time cherished dream of girls and women. I have been seeing patients of hair loss and they would always recall their good days when they used to have good lengthy hair. They would invariably lament about the loss of long hair they were having in teenage and before marriage. This is the type of concern women have for their hair.

Having lusty, shining, long hair is a sign of beauty and feminine grace. Some precautions have to be taken for all types of hair, which are briefed in following heading but long hair need utmost care so that they are not lost easily.

- No brushing should be done immediately after washing.
- Winding the hair, encasing them in rubber bands and then fixing clips or hooks should be done lightly and

never too tightly.

- Winding the hair into tight plaits and then wearing chignon (coil of hair worn at the back of head) pulls the hair from scalp. I have seen many patients, especially girls, having this habit that ultimately ends in bald spots in head.

- Similar is the case with the girls who bind their back hairs in ponytails or buns. One should not confine to one style and go on changing the style so that the hair do not experience a direct pull in this fashion everyday and get pulled.

- Regarding types of curlers, rollers, combs, brushes, etc., these topics are discussed here below under different types of hair. Those rules are applicable for long hair.

Oily Hair

- If you do not apply little amount of oil over the hair regularly, you will loose the hair and their shine.

- The best is to adopt the homeopathic method, 'Like cures like'. Apply little oil to the greasy scalp. Since the scalp itself is producing more of oil, the presence of oil on the scalp would stop production of oil from within. The imbalance will thus be overruled.

- If you are washing the hair twice in a week (women), make it thrice a week. Apply some oil, massage it into scalp and leave it for at least one hour on your scalp before washing it with shampoo. Men should do it five times a week.

- If you are using harsh, highly scented and strong hair-care products like soaps, shampoos and oils, leave them.

- Improve your diet to make it nutritional.

- Take half a bottle of distilled water and add some lemon juice in it. Now rinse your hair with this mixture to remove oiliness of hair.
- It is always in your own interest that you should consult a beauty parlor when you do not find relief after testing the mentioned methods. No relief means that you need help of a conditioner to remove/rectify oiliness.

Dry Hair

- Use of heat- styling appliances; dryers for drying the hair after washing and over-exposure to the sun should be avoided.
- Take nutritional food.
- Do not adopt rigorous cleaning methods or routine.
- Use a good hair oil to massage the hair. If the dryness is more, the hair become brittle. Do not massage the scalp vigorously.
- Steaming the hair once a fortnight also help in dry hairs. Massaging and steaming as a follow-up gives good result.
- Do not wash the hair frequently with shampoo.
- Do not comb or brush strongly.

Use of Home Made Shampoos for Different Kinds of Hair
Oily and Dry Hair

- For oily hair, some toning lotions are available in the market and beauty parlors but if you are interested to try home made shampoos or washers, nothing can compare this home made variety.
- The best is to wash your hair with 'Shikakai' powder and grinded 'methi' powder (fenugreek) in 1:0.25 ratios,

after mixing with white of an egg. This mixture or type of home-made shampoo is for **oily hairs**.

- Another home-made shampoo **for oily hair** is 'Reetha' (dry soap nuts) and 'Shikakai'. Soak 'Reetha' overnight, mash them in the morning and filter it. Now add some 'Shikakai' powder in it, mix it and wash your hairs.

- For **oily hairs,** make a paste of 'Mehndi' powder and curds and apply on the hair. Let it dry for about thirty minutes and then wash the hairs. It is a good conditioner for oily hair.

- For **dry hair,** the mixture is 'Shikakai' and coconut milk. Take a cup of coconut milk and four tea-spoonful of 'Shikakai' and mix them. Apply the paste on the hair, massage the hair and scalp and leave the mixture to dry for five to ten minutes. Now rinse it out.

- Glycerin is a good oily substance. Mix one tea-spoonful of it with some good shampoo available in the market. Now add one tea-spoonful each of castor oil and vinegar. Apply this mixture on **dry hair** and leave them to dry for about 15-20 minutes before rinsing with fresh water.

- There are some **'henna conditioners'** available in the market. They are useful for both dry and oily hair. You can make one at home. One table-spoonful of powder 'Mehndi', one table-spoonful of 'Amla' powder, one table-spoonful of 'Brahmi' or coconut oil and six table-spoonful of luke warm milk. Make a paste of all these ingredients. Apply this paste on the hair and leave it for 30 minutes and then wash the hair. This mixture is useful for **dry hair.**

- 'Amla' oil, glycerin, castor oil, malt vinegar, white of egg and shampoo (any good brand); all these are to be mixed in one tablespoonful quantity. Massage the mixture for five minutes and then rinse the hair with fresh water. This is a good conditioner both for **dry** and **oily hair.**

Wavy Hair (Hairs Having Waves)

- Wavy hair are not curly but have waves as you find in the sea or sand dunes.
- Those who have wavy hair, they should wash their hair with a shampoo that has shine enhancing gradients.
- After washing, dry the hair in natural ways and separate the hair with comb that has wide-teeth so that there is no entanglement and pulling while combing the hair.
- Wavy hair need good conditioners and more care than straight hair.

Straight Hair

- Straight hair lie flat on the scalp.
- Since such hair lie flat, they gather more dust. Naturally these straight hair are mostly dense and hence they need deep cleaning shampoo.
- Such hair need at least three washings a week.
- They are more prone to develop dandruff.
- Oiling and massaging the scalp is essential and it should be one night before washing schedule.

Curly Hair

- Curly hair get dry very soon.
- For washing curly hair, a shampoo with good moisture-gradient is necessary.
- To bring a shine to curly hair, dry them with towel and

expose to sun or natural air. In curly hairs, fingers reach easily up to the scalp. Use your fingers to disentangle them and then use wide toothed comb or brush to keep them at place.

Selection of Hair Oil

It is said that the best hair oil to be used is the one that you have been using since your childhood. If mustard oil is used, continue its application throughout life. If coconut oil is used, keep it applying on the hair althrough the life. This is one aspect over which everyone agrees. There is no need to change the oil. If you go on changing oils, there will be damage to the structure of hair. In cold regions, people use mustard oil and in hot or medium hot regions, coconut oil is best to use. Besides these two, if someone is using 'Amla' (Emblica officinalis) hair oil, it is one of the best oil for hair-health. 'Amla' oil is preferably used in hot and mild hot regions.

There are many branded hair oils available in the market and these are sold with different slogans like cool effect giving, shine enhancing, brain tonic, etc. One should read the contents of the oil before being purchasing. *Oils produced by homeopathic medicine manufacturers* contain Arnica, Jaborandi, Amla, Shikakai, Cantharis, Calendula, etc. in different form with base of coconut or some other oil. Most of the homeopathic hair oils available in the market are named as Arnica hair oil. Arnica is only one of the gradients in the oil.

There are *ayurvedic hair oils* available in the market and they are very popular. These oils contain 'Bhirgraj' (Eclipta alba), 'Amla' (Emblica off.), 'Manjishtha' (Rubia cordifolia), 'Mandukparni' (Centella asiatica), 'Jatamansi' (Nardostachys jatamansi), 'Musta' (Cyperus rotundus), 'Khus' (Vetiveria zizaniodes), 'Gulab' (Rose), 'Pudina phool' (Menthol),

'Karpoor' (Camphor), 'Kapoor-kachri' (Hedychium spicatum) etc. A combination of these herbs are used and mixed with coconut oil as a base and the quantity of herbs also vary. These oils are given different branded names.

Mustard oil mixed with 'Amla' oil is another branded oil available in the market. It may be good for those who have been using mustard or 'Amla' oil in the past. Key ingredients are mustard and 'Amla' in it. This means there are some other scents or secret formula substances also in it. One can use this and find out the results by themselves.

Many oils have been given name with 'cool' effect and these are flooding the market these days under different branded names. The key ingredients in these types of cool oils are 'Menthol' or 'Pudina' oil, 'Chandan' oil, 'Amla' extract, camphor, perfume in mineral or vegetable oils.

The general method of their use is to try these branded oils when one feels that his or her hair are diseased and need help of some oil as claimed by the manufacturer. Any type or brand of one particular oil can be tried for a week and if it favors, this can be continued till the hair falling, dandruff or other diseased condition is cured. Once it is done with, one should return to his or her normal hair oil that had been used prior to the disease.

Massaging / Tugging / Exercises

Massaging the hair means inducing extra life to the health of your hair. It improves the blood circulation of the scalp. A daily massage of ten to fifteen minutes will stimulate the circulation of blood in the scalp. It improves looks of hair, make them strong and reduces the falling of hair.

- Divide your hair into three parts making bunches of hair

together and then separating them into three parts. Now apply hair oil with the help of cotton all along the line of separating hair. Such a division of hair should mean that the oil has been applied all over the scalp.

• Better than the above application of oil with cotton is dipping the finger tips in oil (coconut oil, olive oil or mustard oil, whichever you have been using) and applying oil on the scalp.

• Work your fingers (knuckles) in circular motion on the scalp, forehead, and temples and back of your head. Move the fingers in clockwise and anti-clockwise direction.

• The massage has to be done with gentle strokes in the first instance and then, at times tap the fingers on the scalp with slightly hard strokes.

• Dip your fingers in a tablespoonful of caster oil and let the hair be smoothened with it. Leave the oil for two hours in the hair and then shampoo. You will get a beautiful shine in the hair and it will also seal split ends.

• Applying oil on the scalp and leaving it overnight is also good. Wash the hair in the morning.

• One has to take care that massaging is not too harsh or vigorous. During massaging, some people pull their hair (tugging of hair). This practice is not good as it may damage the hair roots.

• Tugging of hair is a technique different from massaging. It should not be tried at home and help of a professional should be preferred, if tugging is desired.

• After the massaging is over, conduct some neck exercises. Turn you neck to left and then to right, two to three times. Now turn your neck up and down in the same fashion and finally rotate your head in circular motion, clockwise and anti-clockwise. (For complete details of neck exercises, please refer my book, 'Manage and Cure Neck Pain' (B. Jain Publishers).

- Yoga helps to maintain very good overall health of not only hair but also whole body. 'Sheershasan' and 'Sarvangasan' are some of the 'asana' considered best for the health of hairs. 'Sheershasan' is standing on head. 'Sarvangasan'is lying on upper back, supporting loins with hands and raising legs above. While the upper portion of body with shoulders and head are on the ground, the legs are in the air. Both 'asanas' require guidance of a Yoga expert. If you have hypertension or any cardiac problem, do not conduct these 'asanas'.

Selection of Shampoos

Beauty experts prohibit use of bath soaps and advise use of shampoos only. It may be noted that in Indian market, some soaps have been manufactured instead of shampoos. These soaps are made exclusively for washing hair which suit many women. One can try these soaps and if they suit well, there is no need for use of shampoos.

Varieties of shampoos are available in the market and each product has different kind of ingredients. Most of the products claim that their shampoo is herbal based. Word, *herbal,* has become a craze of the trading community. Any product having even a single herb is declared herbal. The amazing part of this trade game is that USA and other Western countries now trade herbs belonging to Indian soil. Recently a big USA firm has launched three kinds of packs called 'herbal' packs for hair, cholesterol and strength with a trade name. They are very costly. The herbal beauty packs marketed by any big Indian firm are equally costly. One should not be misled or confused by 'herbal' contents and check the ingredients of the product before use.

There is very popular oil marketed in India by some name (Not disclosed for obvious reasons) that claims removal of baldness and make rich hair growth. A small bottle of about fifty milliliter costs more than two hundred rupees or so. I am not sure about its worth but people buy it and must be finding good results otherwise the company would have been closed by now.

There are different shampoos for dry, oily or natural hair. Use of shampoo or soap can be decided after their performance on the type of hair individually. Soaps that are mildly scented and bland (their lather do not irritate eyes) are better. In a branded herbal shampoo made by an USA company for normal to oily hair, the stated used gradients are as follows:

Sodium chloride, Sodium laureth sulphate, Cocamide DEA, Cocamidopropyl betaine, water, Fragrance, DMDM hydantoin, Citric acid, Tetrasodium EDTA, Propylene glysol, Chamomile extract, Passion flower extract, Thyme extract, D and C Orange no 4, D and C red no 33, and D and C violet no 2. This is obligatory in USA and other advance countries to write full prescription of gradients in the products for the knowledge of users.

This rule is applicable in India too but the companies find it convenient to write only key-gradients in the products. In one popular brand of Indian shampoo meant for hair fall control, there are only two key-gradients mentioned in the manual provided with the product. These are *Ammonium lauryl sulfate and Ammonium laureth sulfate.*

Another Indian shampoo (herbal) made for dandruff, following gradients are stated in the user's manual: *Rosmaninus officinalis, Azadirachta indica (neem), Ocimum sanctum (tulsi), Acacia concinna (shikakai), Phyllanthus embica (amla) and Lawsonia inemis (henna).*

Instead of shampoo, 'Multini Mitti' can be used for washing the hair. This 'mitti' is available in the market in packets. There

are also shampoos available in the market that have *Aloe vera,
vitamin 'E'* or wild flower in them.

Homeopathic drug manufacturers are also marketing
certain branded shampoos and oils for the care of hair. These
homeopathic shampoos, soaps and oils are useful but it would
have more impact if homeopathic medicines were also taken
with external applications. There is one homeopathic product
(oil, shampoo) of some Kolkata company that provides some
internal medicine also with the pack. I am not sure about the
results but as a rule, it should term better.

The 'so called' homeopathic shampoos have key- gradients
like 'Amla', 'Shikakai', 'Reetha', 'Cantharidin sulphide',
'Arnica montana', 'Calendula' and 'Jaborandi'. As a matter of
fact, this shampoo is a mixture of homeopathic medicines and
ayurvedic medicines. Every product has its specific formula
having two or three medicines from the above list.

- Texture of hair decides the type of soap and shampoo,
  one should use. You can try one shampoo and see the
  results. Try another brand next time and then compare
  the results with the first one. You will know which
  shampoo is best suited to your hair. After this trial, do
  not change brand of shampoo. The contents in the
  shampoo must be read before buying the shampoo. If it
  has been fortified with hair nourishing medicinal herbs,
  it is good.
- Do not shampoo your hair everyday. Shampoo washes
  away dirt is known to all but very few know that frequent
  use of shampoo washes away the hair's protective oils also.
- Frequency of washing of hair depends upon the climate
  and also upon the length of hair.
- When the hair are wet, allow them to dry in their natural
  way.

- Never do brisk rubbing of hair with a towel to dry them up. Sit under a fan, in summer and under a sun, in winter.
- Use of hard shampoos containing chemicals take away the natural oil from the scalp and it should be avoided.
- Shampoos that produce excessive lathering may have excessive percentage of detergents and should be avoided.
- Shampoos that are extremely scented should be avoided. Mildly scented shampoos are supposed to be better.
- It is difficult to select a suitable shampoo for the hair. Do not go by the advertisements on TV and newspapers; use your skill of checking with the ingredients of the shampoo. There are various types of shampoos available in the market labelled as useful for oily or dry hair, useful for dandruff or useful for normal hair and so on. You have to check the actual chemicals in the shampoo.
- Therapeutic shampoo will carry the name of the chemical. Many shampoos meant for dandruff, contain *selenium sulphide and buffered emulsion* to prevent dandruff. Selenium works on the dead debris and slows down their production.
- The important thing is that you should not use this (selenium) shampoo every day. Selenium is a medicine and everyday use of it is not recommended. Overuse of selenium may dry your hair and make them brittle.
- Use other normal shampoos in between two washings of selenium shampoo, say in a week. After use of selenium sulphide shampoo for a month or two, if this is not removing the dandruff, it is better to switch over to other shampoos meant for dandruff.

- Shampoos for dandruff have ingredients like *salicylic acid, sulphur, coal tar, and pyrithione zinc*, etc. You can try them for a limited period and check the results for suitability.
- In case, you find difficulty in selection of the shampoo, consult a dermatologist for a prescription of shampoo.
- The best use to take from shampoo is to leave the shampoo applied on the hair for at least three to four minutes before you rinse out.

WASHING OF HAIR

People living in remote villages of India wash their hair with ordinary bath soaps. In villages or small towns, shampoo pouches are used for washing hair but this is also limited in few families, who are literates, had been to cities and have funds to spend. Women in most of the villages use 'Multani Mitti' (a kind of clay) for washing their hair and it is supposed to be very good conditioner and washing agent. Similarly, use of curds for washing hair is common in villages. Curd is a conditioner as well a remedial measure against falling of hair and dandruff. Curd brings shine in the hair. Use of 'Shikakai, Reetha and Amla' is also a common remedial measure for falling of hair and dandruff in village folks. Henna is widely used as a conditioner and dyeing agent in villages and cities. Efficacy of all these products has to be believed in because they are time-tested and are being used by majority of women. I say majority of women because seventy to eighty percent of our people live in villages.

Get the Washing Effect on Hair Within Minutes

If you are a busy person and could not adhere to your routine of washing the hair with shampoo or if you are not well or had just recovered from a sickness in which doctor has advised you not to wet your hair and you feel that you must get that washed-look on your hairs, here is a trick that would give your hair a temporary shine without shampoo-washing. Sprinkle some talcum powder on the comb and then comb your hairs. Repeat this application of powder on comb and combing for three to four times till you get the said effect, 'as if washed'.

USE OF CONDITIONERS

The conditioning is a procedure of attaching a sort of fixer on the hairs so that the peeling is removed and the hair shaft returns to normal strength. A conditioner can be called a shine enhancer for the hair, which is supposed to improve the texture of hair so that the hair are easily manageable. Conditioners are generally used after shampoo of the hair.

- When the hair become dry, the cuticles (hair shaft, outer layer) come out/peel off from central shaft of hair.
- Many types of conditioners are available in the market and one should select a good conditioner.
- There are conditioners by which you can directly wash the hair and the hair get the required conditioning.
- There are conditioners, which will have to be kept applied on the hair for some time before rinsing.
- There are also deep conditioners, which are mainly for dry, damaged and brittle hair. Deep conditioners have protein in them and it has to be applied for a longer time.
- You must have seen some products (creams and liquids) on the TV that claim to untangle the locked and frizzed hair. This is a cream or liquid-conditioner that softens the hair to enable smooth combing and brushing.
- The conditioners are available according to the type of

hair, dry or oily.

- Too much frequent use of hair conditioner turns the hair greasy. If the hair are already greasy, apply light conditioners only at the end of hair.

- Egg is good conditioner for dry hair. Use of egg on the hair helps the dry hair to get moist. The procedure is beat a fresh egg in half cup of warm water. Apply this beaten egg on the hair and leave it for ten minutes and then rinse out. Egg conditioner can be applied before shampoo too. Apply the mixture on the hair and leave the same on the hair overnight. Next morning, shampoo the hair.

- Olive oil is also a wonderful conditioner for dry hair. Apply olive oil and massage the scalp. Leave the oil on the scalp for fifteen minutes and wash hair with shampoo. Olive oil is supposed to be best hair oil as per belief of people of Greece.

- Sour curd is an excellent hair conditioner that makes the hair softer and brings back the shine. It also stops falling of hair. Apply sour curd that has been kept for two or three days, on the hair. Let it remain on the hair for at least half an hour and then rinse the hair clean of curds.

- Use of olive oil on the hair and then steaming the hair makes the hair shine. Olive oil should be applied on the scalp and after about fifteen minutes, steam the hair by wrapping a towel that has been dipped in hot water. It will give a good conditioning to the hair.

DRYING OF HAIR

- Let the hair dry in natural way and do not use hair dryer. Heat contributes to drying of hair, which is not required.
- In winter, sit in the sun for some time.
- In summer, sit under the fan air for some time.

- Do not use hair dryer, heated rollers or curling wands, for too long and never blow the hot air too near to your hair and scalp.
- Place a dry towel (absorbing Turkish towel) covering the back so that the hair rest on the towel and absorb water.

MAKING HAIR CURLY

- Heat is needed to make hair curly. Better not to use the electric curlers or curling irons.
- If curling of hair is a must, use plastic cylindrical rollers. There are sponge rollers also available in the market that is used to sleep with, at night. Curling can also be done with steam producing heated rollers that are thermostatically controlled.
- The rollers can also be used for straightening the hair by moistening the rollers.
- Perming, bleaching does harm to the hair and scalp.

Note :

Curling of hair should be got done from professionals and if curling is tried at home, it should be strictly according to the instructions of the manufacturers of products being used.

TYPES OF BRUSHES AND COMBS

- If your hair are thick, you will need a soft brush that has soft bristles. Use a comb that has wide teeth space between each tooth.
- If you have light hair, your brush may have flat bristles. The comb may be multi-purpose that have both wide-spaced teeth and narrow spaced teeth on one comb.

- Plastic combs should be avoided because their teeth have sharp edges that can pull the hair out easily. Combs need not be hard. It is preferred to use either rubber combs or wooden combs or combs made out of tortoise skin.
- Always wash your brushes and combs regularly in hot water mixed with soap.
- Let the brushes and combs be left in the above mixture for at least two hours before wiping them.
- There are still wire brushes available for cleaning the combs. Before cleaning the combs in the hot water mixture, it is better to clean them with wire brushes.
- Do not brush or comb your hair with brushes or combs that have broken bristles or broken teeth because they will tear the hair shafts.
- There should be separate hair brushes and hair combs for each person in the family. In no cases, brushes or combs of other persons should be used.

Method of Combing and Brushing

- Dry your hair if you have washed them. Hair are weak when they are wet and may fall with strokes of brushes or fine-combs.
- Allow your hair to fall infront your face and to do this you have to bend forward a little.
- Start combing the hair with wide toothed comb from nape of your neck. Stroke them towards the head and then to the end of hair falling before your face.
- Now erect your posture to standing position instead of former bending posture. Make your combing strokes starting from top of your head down to end of hair.
- Standing straight, now part your hair to sides and

comb the top layers with long strokes to the sides. It is better to part your hair with hand after each stroke of comb.

- Now repeat the above procedure of straightening your hair with brush this time.
- It is always better to use combs first before using brushes.
- Combing or brushing of hair should be normally done once or twice in a day.
- No force should be applied while combing and brushing.
- **Finally, never be in a hurry to comb your hair.** Always be patient while combing your hair and adopt above procedure of combing in a very slow manner so that hair do not get entangled and fall. In case you are in a hurry, moist your hair a bit and apply very little glycerin applied on your fingers and then on to the hair. **Some branded gels are available in the market, which claim that hair do not entangle while combing. These can be tried if you are in a hurry.**

USE OF PINS, RUBBER RINGS, CLIPS AND NETS

- If you feel the need to give some style and shape to your hair, there is no harm to use pins, clips, rubber rings and nets.
- These accessories do not bring in any problem of skin provided they are not tightly worn.
- If the clips are of plastic or any other metal except iron, it is better to check for skin allergy. If some rashes or itching comes up after their use, they should be replaced with suitable substance (other than metal).
- While making a pony-tail of hair or winding them by

making knots, it is better not to pull the hair harshly. Insert the rubber rings or clips gently. Constant tension of pulling on the hair may cause hair loss.

- While making the knots or gathering the hair in one hand after removing the already fitted clips or pins, **do not put the pins and clips in your mouth to hold them** temporary for further inserting them in hair. This may infect your mouth if your hair have dandruff or some scalp infection.

- There are no adverse effects of using nets over bunch of hair to make a **'Juda'** and unite them. Keeping a puff or some round soft sponge hidden in the hair to give a shape to 'Juda' is also free of any adverse effect provided it is not heavy and hair do not suffer a pull due to their use.

CARE OF HAIR IN RAINY SEASON

After a spell of hot summer in which hair have to undergo tremendous heat, the rain comes as a relief to the skin. The summer brings in small crop of boils or dandruff on the scalp in some persons and with the onset of rains; all these skin problems get cured of their own without any treatment. This is true in North India. Here, the rains means indigestion, respiratory problems, skin diseases related to fungus including hair diseases. Falling of hair, dandruff and itching of scalp is common in rainy season. If you happen to go to North Eastern states of India, the picture is different so far as the care of hair is concerned. I have been to Assam, Manipur, Nagaland, Meghalaya and Bhutan and observed their culture, living style and traditions. The ladies, there, mostly keep short hairs like boys or get their hair trimmed at the end of hair shafts. They cover the heads with variety of hats and scarf so that the hair do not get spoiled due to excessive drenching with frequent hard sunshine. More than five months of intermittent rains in a year in those regions make the hair of the inhabitants strong enough to bear the winds and rains. Their digestion also get adjusted and acclimatized with the season.

To avoid the problems of hair in rainy season one has to be particular about the following:

- Avoid going in the rains and sun heat during spells of rains. Otherwise, cover your hair.
- Take your meals in time and try to take balanced nutrient food.
- Include foods having proteins ('Channa, Rajma, Soyabean', Cheese, etc.), take fruits that are seasonal.
- Better not to take milk in rainy season. Reduce intake of curds also.
- Take buttermilk instead of milk and curds.
- Protect your head from getting drenched in rains but if you get wet, better dry your hair at the earliest.
- Do not take foods that have lot of spices.
- Give a massage of coconut oil on your scalp every third day during rainy season. This massage should be done at night and hair should be washed in the morning.
- One should go to sleep early and avoid watching TV late at night. Get up early in the morning. These habits bring heat in the head that spoils the health of hairs.
- During rainy season, do not wash your hair with soap. Wash your hair with 'Multani mitti'.
- Deficiency of calcium and iron also bring in hair falling in rainy season. Take juice of lemon, amla, honey, apple, banana, tomatoes and oranges from time to time.
- If you catch cold in rainy season, get this treated at the earliest. A prolonged cold harms the hair.

PROTECTION OF HAIR
Protection of Hair from Storms, Rains and Sun

- Hair on the head are hangings or lying strands of threads, a sort of fabric and need due protection.
- If the hair are exposed to high velocity winds and rains, their strength of holding the scalp gets weak.
- The dirt gathered in the hair due to storms or pollution in the air should be washed after storms and rains.
- The hair will tend to fall before their stipulated time of natural falling, if they are frequently exposed to winds. It is better to wear a head cover in such seasons.
- In the sun heat, the hair absorb excessive heat and tend to fall. A hair covering is necessary.
- Similar is the condition of hair in winters when snow falls or there is fog or frost in the air.
- Better wear a scarf or hat during the storms, sunny days, foggy days and rains.

Protection of Hair when Taking Bath in Swimming Pools

- Water in the swimming pools has an additive called chlorine, which is not good for the health of hair.
- Before entering the swimming pool, apply and rub some coconut oil or mustard oil, whatever you have been using.
- While taking a bath in swimming pool, better use a rubber cap.
- Oil application will provide an extra protection in case the water enters the hair in spite of wearing the cap.

ROUGH IDEA ABOUT COST OF HAIR AND BODY CARE IN BEAUTY CLINICS (DELHI)

	Rupees
Hair cut (Plain dry)	75 to 100
Blow dry	75 to 100
Ironing	100 to 150
Crimping	150 to 200
Shampoo (including plain dry)	25 to 50
Henna	75 to 125
Oil massage head, coconut	75 to 125
Oil massage head, olive oil	100 to 150
Full body massages (coconut, olive, aroma and anti cellulite)	250 to 500
Deep hair conditioning	150 to 200
Straightening hair	750 to 800
Hair color	800 to 900
Streaking	1,000 to 1200
Perming	700 to 800
Waxing (full, arms and legs)	150 to 200
Arms full	50 to 75
Legs full	75 to 100
Bleach, face and neck	75 to 200
Body bleach	475 to 500
Hair microwefting	3,000 to 10,000 (depending upon the area.)

□□□

Chapter 7
Styles of Hair
---

1. INTRODUCTION
2. HAIR FIXERS
3. COMBS, BRUSHES, AND ROLLERS FOR STYLING
4. PERMING OF HAIR
5. NATURAL CURLY HAIR

Styles of Hairs

INTRODUCTION

Every one desires a different hair style to look different from others and appear beautiful. Hair style is done by beauty parlors according to the shape of face.

If some one is having an oval / long face and straight hair, the person will look awful. The hair stylist would like to give the straight flat hair a puffy or round style so that the length of face looks short.

If you observe the hair styles of actors and actresses of films, you will realize that they change the style according to the character played by them. In the early sixties, when the fashion of styling the hairs was not much in vogue, actors and actresses had developed a unique style. Devanand had a style that showed a bunch of hairs elevated on one side of head. Dilip Kumar had rough wandering hairs with a group of strands decorating forehead. This style can be seen now on the head of actor Shahrookh Khan. Raj Kapoor, the actor had wavy hair-style and Shammi Kapoor used to wear long hair curling on forehead. Sadhna had a hairstyle, which fixed hair on her forehead in a straight line parallel to eyebrows. This style was named as 'Sadhna hair cut' and it is in the latest trends today. Famous TV character 'Jassi' wears the same style. Those who have seen film actress Mumtaz of the seventies must have noted her 'side-flick' hairstyle. The same style has come back and can be seen in TV serial 'Kahani ghar ghar ki' where character Parvati and her daughter Shruti wear the same 'side flicks' hair style.

The hair style is maintained to fix the hair in shape and create new looks. In the olden days, there were popular brands of hair creams and fixers available in the market, which claimed fixation of hair in any style by their application.

Today many styling creams and other products or tools are available in the market. Different hair style are in fashion and beauty parlors help in styling the hair as one desires. Hair styling infuses confidence in the person and he or she feels elevated in personality.

Following is the list of products available in the market for styling. It is better if professionals and beauty parlors do the styling of hair so as to achieve good results.

Shape of Face, Height and Style Relationship

The hair style is directly related to the shape of face and height. A proportion and relationship has to be maintained in hair style and the shape of head. This can be adequately proved that only long, dense hair do not decorate the personality of a lady, if she is of less than normal height and if her face is oval type. In such person, the long hair cannot be left hanging. They will look odd. The hair have to be styled in widening form so that oval or long face looks normal. Actually it is the shape of jaws that decides the shape of face and hence locks of hairs or bundles of hair are to be centered on jaws. A professional hair stylist can decide the type of hair which you should wear. Here are some recommended hair styles in short:

Long Face
(U type jaws) The hair should be placed in such a fashion that they do not add more height on the head. The hair may have a wide spread lay-out on the forehead.

Round face
(Circular jaws) Hair on the head may be placed flat and on the sides of face, they should fall on both the cheeks to hide the rounded face.

Square face
(Square jaws) Hair to be kept in such a fashion that adds some width overlapping the ends of jaws.

Triangular face
(Pointed chin) Some branches of hair are to be spread on the forehead so that length of the face hides.

HAIR FIXERS
Creams or Balms
Creams and balms help in holding the hair in the desired fashion, be it straight, curled or puffed. These creams tame the unmanageable flying hairs and also handle short and lengthy hair at one area in position. All you have to do is to wet your

hair by spraying water and then drench the hair with cream or balm through play of fingers and combs / brushes. Set them in desired direction and they will remain in the same position till you wash the hair.

Hair sprays

Hair sprays have been in use since last fifty years or so in India and are very popular. There are mainly three types of hair sprays available in the market.

1. **Pump type spray** is used by pumping the handle of the bottle (mechanical). They take longer time to get dry because they tend to be wet due to unequal pressure of hand while spraying.

2. **Aerosol type spray** is also mechanical since it needs pressure of finger but the spray is through pressure of air or gas. This spreads the spray of fixing-liquid in all direction in a finer way. The spray dries quickly and with ease to settle the hair in desired fashion.

3. **Freezing spray** is available in both pump and aerosol containers and when sprayed, they hold the hair very firmly. They are meant where hard and firm hair shapes and moulds are needed.

Gels

As the name indicates, gels are in semi-liquid form. They are available in thick, heavier or light as per the need of the customer. Thick and heavy gels are used to straighten the hair. The light gels are in liquid form and used for smoothening the hair so that they do not entangle. Many of you must have seen advertisement on TV about easy disentangling of hair after bath by use of some particular brand of liquid. It is this light gel. Gels are capable of creating a wet look in the hair and on drying; the desired shape can be given to the hair. The same is done by again wetting the hair a little.

Pomades

Pomades are used to control the texture of curly hair. It is better not to use the pomade on light and fine hair growths because the pomade itself is heavy and it will weigh down the hair and they would look scarce. Use of pomade brings shine to the hair besides setting and styling the hair.

Volumizers

Volumizers, as the name indicates, act to give the hair a look as if there is a great volume of hair on the head. It is mostly in spray form but available in lotions also. Its use sets the different shaft of hair together so that the hair give a thicker and fuller look. Those who have flat hair that keep on lying on the scalp use this product.

COMBS, BRUSHES, AND ROLLERS FOR STYLING

The combs, rollers and brushes play a great role in styling the hair at home. While combing can be done on wet hair, brushes and rollers cannot be used on wet hair. Combs should also be used on slightly wet hair so that they do not get entangled or pulled.

Brushes

- Brushes are best style makers than combs. After the use

of wide-teeth combs, it is the turn of brushes to style the hair.

- Brushes and combs stimulate the blood circulation of scalp and enhance supply of natural oil from root to the end of hair.
- Plastic brushes with somewhat round balls at the end of tooth gives smooth and gentle caressing to the scalp.
- Plastic brushes with full round bristles all over its circumference are available in many diameters. Those having narrow diameter are better for hair styling.
- Plastic brushes with half round bristles are not for styling but for simple brushing when you are in hurry to dress up your hair.
- Brushes with flat, plastic or nylon bristles are useful when brushing is needed after drying the hair. These brushes are also useful for erasing dandruff or scaling.

Rollers

- **Plastic rollers** are meant for making curls on the hair provided they are short in length.
- **Hot rollers** are used for making hair curly. They are available in three sizes, large, medium and small and they are used on dry hair only.
- **Velcro rollers** are very easy to use because no pins are needed to hold them in places. They are used on dry hair for quick setting and curling.
- **Cushioned rollers** are of great use when the rolling / curling / setting of hair is done overnight, while sleeping.
- **Steam rollers** are useful for all types of hair. They are

smooth and gentle on the hair when they wrap and can give good curly hair. They are thermo-controlled.

Blow Dryers and Iron

- Blowers or blow dryers are good tools for styling the hair. These dryers are easily available in small and big cities.
- Dryers are of two types. **Dryer with brushing facility** brush the hair while drying.
- Dryer with **long nozzle fit-in** has an edge over the brush dryers since it gives good flexibility in styling.
- Diffusers (an attachment) are available to be fitted with dryers. It is attached to the nozzle of dryer to disperse heat evenly across broad sections of hair, while leaving curls in tact.
- Some beauty parlors use irons to give a style to the hair. This technique is not healthy for hair and can damage the hair due to direct heat application on the strands of hair. This may also cause burns. Preferably, irons should not be used on hair.

Shaping / Cutting Hair with Flame or Iron without the use of Scissors

With term 'burns', let me tell you about the latest trend of beauty parlors to do a hair cut and shape them into a style *without the use of scissors*. Some beauty parlors in USA, European countries and India have started burning the hair ends to make them short and stylish. They do not use scissors to cut the hair short but use naked flame or irons to burn the hair short from their ends. The experts in hair styling and in business of saloons do not recommend this technique of cutting short the hair as healthy. Although there is no residue / dirt of cut- hairs

F- 13

on the clothes or body when trimmed with heaters yet the heat of fire from stem, shaft to root is not supposed to be healthy for the scalp.

However, if some people like the heat method for cutting hair short, wavy or curly, it is always better to get it done from experts. There are many types of irons used for different purposes. They are corkscrew irons, bristled irons, crimpling irons and basic curling irons.

PERMING OF HAIR
(PERMANENT ARTIFICIAL WAVES)

- Making artificial curls in the hair in a permanent way is called perming. Perming is normally well done in the beauty parlors and saloons under the guidance of expert cosmetologists.
- The curls in the hair are done by means of lotions, rollers, perm solutions, fixer rods and wrappings. By this method, the hair curl is permanently waved in the hair.
- This cannot be destroyed by shampoo washing or oiling but the curls can get a little relaxed.
- For washing the hair, there are special shampoos available that are meant for use after perming.
- It is advised that permed hair should not be washed up to 48 hours of perming.
- The perming never fades completely and goes only after a haircut. The hair would grow straight, as were they before perming.
- Once the perms in the hair are cut, they would require further perming treatment, if so desired.
- The accessories and perming solutions are available in the market and if perming is done at home, it would need lot of experience and there is possibility of damage

to the hair by the use of chemicals, which are applied in proper ratio. If this ratio is not maintained properly, damage to the hair is sure. It is therefore desired that the job of perming should be under the guidance of experts in beauty parlors. It takes about 2 to 3 hours time to get the whole job of perming done.

- If a hair cut is desired, it should be done prior to perming. If you get the hair-cut done after perming, there is likelihood of hair getting straight after the perms are cut.
- Drier should not be used frequently to dry the permed hair. They should be dried in natural way.
- Perming remains on the hair for four to six months and depends upon the nature of lotion and technique applied while perming.

NATURAL CURLY HAIR

In South India, people have more of curly hair than people in North India. People living in coastal areas also have curly hair as compared with people living away from coasts. For ladies having curly hair, there is less of scope for different styles of hair. The irony is that ladies having curly hair desire their hair flat and those having flat hair desire curly hair.

- If you desire to straighten your curly hair, it should be got done from beauty parlors that iron them. Ironing would make them straight till you wash them. After washing curl return. It is, therefore, unnecessary to get the curly hair straightened except on special occasions when the ladies want so temporary.
- Those who have curly hair by nature, they have little option for hair-cuts and change in style.
- They can either cut the hair short or keep very lengthy

hair. Short hair would look less curly and long hair would look flat. Lengthy hair can be wrapped and a ponytail can be made for a style. Still if some style in curly hair is needed, the best way is to get them colored in different streaks.

- Curly hair need washing twice a week.
- People having curly hair should use those shampoos, which are meant for dry hair.
- If the hair are already curly and more of artificial perms are needed for better style, this can also be done by the professionals.
- Application of hair pack containing 'Multani mitti' is good for curly hair to give them shine.

Homeopathy in Treatment of Hair Problems

Chapter 8

Homeopathy in Treatment of Hair Problems

INTRODUCTION

Irrespective of treatment of hair diseases, one must know the system of homeopathy first. There are certain rules to be obeyed. The students, doctors and followers of homeopathy must have preliminary knowledge about homeopathy. Here is a recollection of this system of medicine that you might have already read. This book has been written for all irrespective of their knowing homeopathy or not. Please bear with me if you know all the facts written below. You may even shift over or skip to next pages to find your choice of therapy. Those who are interested in homeopathy can continue reading.

Those who have experienced the cures of homeopathy always adore this system of medicine. Those who have not tried homeopathy have many misleading views and concepts about this therapy. With homeopathy lingers a puzzling stigma as to whether it really works or not? Is homeopathy an ardent belief that has no rational scientific proof ? Is it a trial people give when allopathy fails to cure a disease? In the whole world, India ranks first in advocating and practicing homeopathy. Homeopathy is not only popular in cities but in remote villages of eastern India. Today there are *172 teaching institutes (UG) and 24 PG faculties in India. There are 307 hospitals and 7411 dispensaries. The number of registered medical practitioners in homeopathy is about two lakhs.* This shows that the system has something in its root and people are drawn towards it. The big question still remains in the air. Does it work? Is it reliable? These doubts have not come overnight. First, homeopathy is not considered a scientific system in many countries and even in India, there are people who do not believe in its therapeutic value. Secondly, it has limitations in surgical cases, handling heart disease in emergency, meeting requirements of accident cases, acute epidemic diseases, severe painful attacks and so on. Such evanesce of a major physical plight make homeopathy vulnerable.

Most of the people depend upon allopathic treatment although tens of other systems of medicine exist. Allopathy handles all types of diseases and cure is said to be quick. Ayurveda, unani, homeopathy, acupuncture, magneto therapy, pranic healing, reiki and others therapies take time to cure and their doctors or chemists are not readily available in all towns or cities. These therapies cannot handle emergencies, injuries, accidents and severe cardiac problems. On the other hand, allopathic doctors and hospitals are at our doorsteps. In spite of this, the irony is that general antagonism against 'Angrezi dawa' exists for its adverse side- effects. People, therefore, wish to switch to other therapies provided they are educated about them. In recent times, homeopathy has gained heights for its no side effects and cheaper cost of treatment. Its 'drawbacks' are stated to be delayed cure, limitations in accidents and tackling severe cardiac problems. Its capacity to cure warts, moles, scars, kidney stones and benign tumors is known. Allopathy resorts to surgery for this. Homeopathy has worldwide reputation for 'Calcarea phos.', the medicine to help teething. Even allopathic doctors prescribe Calcarea phos. these days. Homeopathy can be made use of, provided we have adequate knowledge about it. Let us explore potential of homeopathy for its maximum utilization.

WHAT IS HOMEOPATHY?

It is a system based upon a fixed principle, 'Similia similibus curenture' or 'like cure like'. This means a diseased organ needs a drug that can create similar symptom of the disease a man suffers from. For instance, Ipecacuanha (a herb) when taken in crude form has quality of creating vomiting but when an ailing man suffering from vomiting takes homeopathically prepared Ipecacuanha, the vomiting stops. Dr. C.F. Samuel Hahnemann conceived this principle in 1790 when he was translating Cullen's materia medica. He was basically a qualified allopathic doctor of the times. He chanced upon an observation about cinchona having healing properties for malaria. He took this drug, although he was not suffering from malaria. He was surprised that he developed malaria fever symptom. This is how homeopathy was born. He undertook many more experiments and proved many medicines upon himself. In 1806, he published his first book, 'Medicine of experience', a precursor of the 'Organon', called 'GITA' of homeopathy. It is now a basic theory book on homeopathy.

Proving of drugs was the prime job for Hahnemann. He selected his curative agents (medicines) from four kingdoms, the man, the animal, the vegetable and the minerals. He professed that rational doctrine of therapeutics begins with the changes brought about in a man. These changes are called symptoms. His theory was thus based upon symptoms-observation without any reference to the name of disease. The best way to observe symptoms was an epidemic where symptom could be viewed collectively as an unit. This brought in totality of symptoms of particular epidemic-disease. He searched through a cholera epidemic and found resemblance of collective symptoms tallying with mainly three drugs, Cuprum metallicum, Veratrum album and Camphora. He then used these three remedies on healthy persons and noted down the created symptoms. This is how he sized his materia medica initially. Today, we have a long list of proved drugs with some addition by our great Indian doctors who proved Indian herbs. A keen observation of symptom is a must for selecting a single remedy. There are hundreds of medicines for one ailment and it is correct observation of symptoms, which points to ONE remedy out of hundreds. This is the skill of homeopathy.

Vital Force

There is a balancing mechanism in our body that keeps us healthy. This mechanism is called 'vital force' or an energetic entity that has no physical or chemical existence in the body and still it works in our body giving life to us. Homeopathic medicines do not act on diseased organs but on this vital force. Vital force can be compared with endocrinal immunity system or termed as 'defense mechanism' of body. Diseases attack only when vital force is weak. Homeopathic medicines act as catalyst to re-energize the body through gentle stimulation of vital force. The principle that acts in homeopathy is 'Like cures like'. It means that in order to cure disease, we must seek medicines that can excite similar symptoms in the healthy body. Symptoms of the sick person are taken and compared with the symptoms produced by a medicine. If a healthy person takes common salt in excess in his diet for a continuous period, he is likely to have nutritive changes and retention of salt in his body producing dropsy, edema, changes in blood constituents, anemia and leucocytosis. When medicine made out of salt is given to a healthy person, his body will produce similar symptoms as produced by the patient who had been taking excessive salt. When salt in homeopathic form is inducted as a medicine to the person suffering from above symptoms, he is bound to get relief on the principle 'like cures like'. Homeopath has to select such medicine that has similar symptoms as that of a patient. If four patients having fever consult homeopath, they will get four different medicines for same fever because every one has fever with different symptoms. One patient is having tremendous thirst with fever the other has no thirst, one is chilly, the other is hot, one is having headache with fever and the other has vomiting with fever. Only that medicine will be suitable which matches the symptoms of individual patient. A medicine selected for fever with no thirst cannot be given to patient having fever with intense thirst. If some homeopath does not select medicine according to symptoms of the body, failure is on his part and not of the principle of homeopathy. If the selection of remedy is correct, the cure is quick. Homeopathic medicines cure quickly when selection of the medicine is correct.

No Medicine in Homeopathy, is it True?

Many people are of the view that there is no medicine in homeopathic drugs. How is it so? Take example of common salt that is used as a medicine. A drop of salt-water is dissolved in 99 drops of distilled water and shaken/vibrated. The resultant is salt dilution with power (ratio 1 to hundred) of 1c. Now a drop of 1c dilution is taken and mixed with another 99 drops of distilled water and shaken. The outcome is salt dilution with 2c power. This method is repeated to make progressive dilutions of 3c, 4c and so on. When this progressive dilution reaches 12c, there is no atom or molecule of salt in the dilution. It looks like simple water and is named homeopathic medicine, Natrium mur. *This shocks the very basic of homeopathy* because this has been proved adequately in twentieth century through tests like 'high performance liquid chromatography', 'gas liquid chromatography' and 'atomic absorption spectra-photometer' (ASS) that 12c power dilution has no content of medicine. But the position is different now. It is established that matter can be created by annihilation of the mentioned particle into pair of gamma rays by materialization of electromagnetic waves into an electron positron (particle with positive electric charge) pair.

In making of homeopathic medicine (salt here), friction of salt- dilution with walls of phial produces static electricity and creates electromagnetic field. Since frictional- vibrations fluctuate and vary, such variations in electromagnetic field produce electro positron pairs and light isotopes of drug molecules (salt here). More progressive is the dilution (say 30c, 200c, 1000c); more powerful is the drug and contain tremendous healing properties. The light isotopes are capable of penetrating deep into cells of body and even reach genetic level. Now nobody can say that there is no content of medicine in homeopathic remedies. Medical authorities of some countries still doubt about the medicine contents in homeopathic remedies. An open-minded debate is needed to reach conclusion when monitors of conventional systems nurture opposition for homeopathy.

Reactions and Suppressions

It is very much safe and free from reactions provided it is in safe hands and the doctor is experienced. A pioneer of homeopathy, Dr. Kent has said that he would rather share a room with a nest of vipers than be subjected to the administration of medicine from an inexperienced homeopath. If someone takes a wrong medicine over a period of time, there is possibility of proving the medicine. He will suffer from the symptoms, the medicine is supposed to induct and the cure will not be there. It is also unsafe if the patient does the medication by himself without knowledge of homeopathy. I have seen parents giving Calcarea phos. to their children for a continuous period of years. Those who do not know homeopathy prescribe them verbally without telling them the dose and frequency. Over-use of medicine in homeopathy is harmful.

Homeopathic medicines do not cause suppression. Suppression is possible if the doctor prescribes oral medicines (internal intake) and also allows external application of allopathic creams (cortisone for example) in skin diseases. Such an action may eliminate the skin disease temporarily but it will return due to suppression by cream. Poor choice of remedy also leads to suppression.

Placebo Effect

A placebo is a pill without medicine. Some people believe that homeopathic medicines have placebo effect. If you want to check its potential, give it to a person having non-bleeding head injury or earache / toothache. Give placebo and there would not be relief in pains. Homeopaths give placebo after giving high potency medicine (power of medicine like 200c, 1000c). It is to wait for the action of high potency medicine and satisfaction of patient that placebo is used.

Homeopathy is Safe for Children

- When fever, cough, sore throat, cold are in the starting stage.
- When boils, rashes, pimples and other skin diseases are in the initial stage.
- When there are warts, corns and moles on the skin.
- When constipation, diarrhoea, colic, teething occurs.
- When worm affections and bed-wetting is not responding to other system of medicines.
- When injuries are non-bleeding type.

Homeopathy is Safe for Adults

- When obstinate constipation, flatulence, acidity, dyspepsia are recurring complaints.
- When warts, tumors and corns are recommended for surgical removal.
- When skin disorders return after application of ointments is stopped.
- When styes (eruptions over eye lids) and stomatitis (mouth ulcers) is troubling frequently.
- When kidney stones need expulsion, piles need curing and you want to avoid surgery, a chance should be given to homeopathy.
- When nausea and vomiting in pregnancy is not

controlled by other systems of medicine.

- When there is after-effect of vaccinations, surgical operations and teeth extractions.
- When rapid calcification and joining of bones is needed after the fractures of bones and when plastering has already been done.
- When chronic diseases are not getting cured in other system of medicines.

Homeopathy is Not Safe

- When infants are in acute diseased conditions that may endanger their life.
- When severe cuts, injuries and wounds occur.
- When bones are fractured.
- When acute dyspnea (short of breath) is reported that need inhalers or oxygen.
- When dehydration takes place that need intravenous glucose.
- When cardiac problems are significant that need intensive care.
- When epileptic fits or convulsions occur.
- When eye cataract and vision is involved.
- When diabetes, type II or I is involved.
- When retention of urine, strangulation of intestines, hernia or appendix affections are significant.
- When epidemics exist.
- When bleeding from any organ is not getting controlled.
- When gangrene, syphilis and VD is in secondary stage.
- When typhoid, pneumonia, pleurisy and tuberculosis are in second stage.
- When patient is under coma or unconscious.
- When the patients have AIDS or cancer attack.

These are general guidelines and not a definite demarcation between yes and no. One must remember that life of a patient cannot be put to risk when life saving allopathic system is readily available. On the other hand, one must try homeopathy to realize its actual potential.

Homeopathic medicines are very useful in curing diseases of hair but self-treatment of hair diseases is difficult and it is always better to consult a competent homeopath for treatment.

Here is a list of medicines of general use for the knowledge of those who are interested to try these at home. Rest assured these homeopathic medicines are free from any adverse effect and have no reactions.

MEDICINES FOR EACH DISEASE
Rules of Taking Medicines

- Remedies given against each disease or disorder are in the order of preference. First remedy to be given in the first instance failing which the second and then the third one if the second fails.
- All medicines are to be taken in 30th potency.
- 4 pills make a dose.
- The size of pills should be 30.
- Four doses are to be taken in a day at an interval of 3 hours.
- When there is no relief after taking the first medicine for seven days, change to the second remedy and consequently to third remedy finding no relief by again eight doses.
- When there is no relief even after taking all the three medicines turn by turn, consult a homeopath.
- When the relief is complete and immediate after 4

doses, reduce the doses to three the next day and then reduce to two doses on third day and finally one dose a day on fourth day before finally stopping the medicine on eighth day.

- If there is relief by the use of first remedy, there is no need to take second medicine and follow the instructions for reducing the dosage as given in the above paragraph.
- Similarly if the relief comes by use of second or third remedy, follow the above procedure.

Name of Disease/Disorder	Remedies		
	I	II	III
Alopecia (Falling of hair)	Lyc.	Ph-ac.	Wies.
Hair falling after pregnancy and disease	Nat-m.	Sep.	—
Hair on face on lips/chin of women* (*consult a doctor)	Thuj.	Ol-j. 3x	—
Hair falling after parturition	Carb-v.	Sulph.	Lyc.
Hair oily and greasy	Bry.	Merc.	Ph-ac.
Hair dry	Calc.	Thuj.	Sulph.

GENERAL MEDICINES

Note :

Following medicines are to be taken for seven days after which doctor should be consulted. One dose is of four pills and three doses are to be taken in a day.

F- 14

Hair Falling

After acute illness	Carb-v. 30	Three times a day for seven days
After child birth	Lyc. 30	-Do-
After shocks and grief	Ph-ac. 30	-Do-
After injury	Iod. 30	-Do-
After menopause	Sep. 30	-Do-
When combing	Canth. 30	-Do-
At climaxis	Sep. 30	-Do-
Split hair	Thuj. 30	-Do-
In bunches	Calc. 30	-Do-
Hair falling from eyelashes	Rhus-t. 30	-Do-
Too much sweating on hair, falling	Chin. 30	-Do-
During lactation	Nat-m. 30	-Do-
Unruly, sandy, harsh lusterless hair	Sulph. 30	-Do-
Rough, tangling, sticking hair	Borx. 30	-Do-

Dandruff

— White scaly dandruff, dry hair, and falling of hair: *Thuj. 30,* three times a day for seven days. Consult a doctor later.

— With itching and burning or eruptions on scalp: *Graph. 30,* take in the above manner.

— With thick yellow crusts, eczema, and pimples, falling of hair: *Calc. 30,* in the above manner.

— Dandruff in circles like ringworm, moist scalp, and pimples on forehead: *Sep. 30* in the above manner.

— Dandruff with offensive smell: *Psor. 200,* one dose for

one week. Consult doctor later.

— With great itching and loss of hair: *Mez. 30,* three times a day for seven days.

— With nightly burning and itching, dry scales, fair skin patients: *Ars. 30,* in the same above manner.

— White scaly dandruff alternating with cold, sneezing and loss of smell: *Nat-m. 30,* in the same manner.

Gray, Premature Hair

Lyc., Ph-ac., Wies., Graph. and *Thyroid.* are to be tried turn by turn according to symptoms *under the guidance of a doctor.* It takes very long period to cure this disease.

Hair Falling from Different Locations

The medicines given here below are for the reference of doctors only:

— **On forehead** : Ars., Bell., Hep., Merc., Nat-m., Phos., Sil.

— **On Occiput** : Calc., Carbo-v., Hep., Petr., Sep., Sil., Staph., Sul.

— **On sides** : Bov., Graph., Kali-c., Ac-Ph., Sabina., Staph., Zinc.

— **On temples** : Calc.; Kali-c., Lyc., Merc., Nat-m.,

— **On vertex** : Bar-c., Calc., Graph., Hep., Lyc., Nit-. ac., Sel., Sep., Sil., Zinc.

— **On Beard** : Agar., Ambr., Calc., Graph., Nat-m., Nit-ac., Plb., Sil.

— **On moustache** : Bar- c., Kali- c., Plb., Sel.

— **On eyebrows** : Agar., Bell., Caust., Hell., Kali-c., Par., Ph-ac., Plb., Sel.

— In spots, alopecia areata : Ars., Apis, Calc., Canth., Fl ac., Hep., Iod., Lyc., Nat-m., Petr., Phos.

— Falling of eye lashes : Alum., Apis, Aur-, Ars., Petr., Rhus-t.

Falling of Hair—Causation

— **Debility** : Chin.

— **Eczema** : Graph., Kali-bi.

— **Endocrine problems** : Pituin., Thyroid.

— **Fevers** : Fol-ac.

— **Grief** : Ph-ac., Staph.

— **Injury** : Hyper.

— **After chronic headache** : Aloe, Nat-m., Sep.

— **Mental trauma** : Ign.

— **After parturition** : Calc.

— **During menopause** : Lach.

— **During pregnancy and during lactation** : Nat-m.

Last Words

All the hair diseases should preferably be referred to a competent homeopath.

□□□

BIBLIOGRAPHY

Organon of medicine   S.Hahnemann

Chronic diseases   S.Hahnemann

Lectures on Homeopathic   J. T. Kent
   Materia Medica

Repertory of Homeopathic   J. T. Kent
   Materia Medica

Lectures on Homeopathic philosophy   J. T. Kent

Boenninghausen's therapeutic   H.A. Roberts and
   pocket book   Annie C. Wilson

Book of Surgery   Baily and Love

Atlas of Anatomy   Trevor Weston

Comparative Materia Medica   N. C. Ghosh
   and therapeutics

Plain talks on Materia Medica   Willard Ide Pierce
   with comparisons

Homeopathic Materia Medica   W. Boerick
   and Repertory

Chronic miasms and pseudo psora	J. H. Allen
Prescriber	John H. Clarke
Materia Medica	C. Hering
Select your remedy	R. B. Bishamber Das
Homeopathic Prescriber	K. C. Bhanja
Bedside Prescriber	J. N. Shinghal
Science of Homeopathy	George Vithoulkas
Domestic physician	Constantine Herring
Repertory of Homeopathic Nosodes and Sarcodes	Berkley Squire
Concise repertory	S. R. Phatak
Life of Hahnemann	Rosa. W. Hobhouse
Snapshot Prescriber	A. C. Dutta
Su jok Nail Therapy	Park, Jae, Woo
Hair, Skin and Beauty care	Blossom Kochhar
Hair Loss	Farokh J. Master
Hair Care	Kirti Singh
Diseases of hair and nails	Y. R. Aggrawal
Human anatomy and physiology	V. Tatarinov
Essentials of Homeopathic Materia Medica and pharmacy	W. A. Dewey
Practice of Medicine	F. W. Price

Practioner's guide to Gall bladder
  stones and Kidney stones   Shiv Dua

Oral Diseases   Shiv Dua

Neck pain, cervical spondylosis   Shiv Dua

Know and solve your thyroid problems   Shiv Dua

□□□